F

"Dr. Tirrito's approac........se, along with management of cardiac risk factors, has ....ent success for many of my patients. His one-on-one care and comprehensive follow-up is what prevention is all about."

– Jeffrey I. Selwyn, MD

"As a practicing physician, I have found the HeartWise Program extremely effective for my patients. It not only improves their physical health, but also their general well-being."

–Kimberly Carlson, DO

Patient Testimonials

A.R. – "The program works. I've lost almost 45 pounds and feel great!"

C.R. – "Dr. Tirrito's HeartWise program is great! He gives you the tools you need to make positive food and fitness choices."

Y.H. – "Dr. Tirrito starts you out by testing you. You are given your resting heart rate, your caloric intake for the day should be, and whether your metabolic system is working right. It's a very very doable program but the thing that makes it work the best is writing down everything you eat every day. The exercise part is great too. He helps you increase your exercise. It needs a balance. He wants me cardiac healthy as well as weight healthy. I do tell everyone about the program."

R.H. – "It's not easy. It takes work. The hardest part for me is exercise. My ankles don't hurt anymore when I walk. I'm down 66 pounds and have another 26 more pounds to go."

M.M.G. – "It's been wonderful. I have lost a total of 74 pounds so far. He's very encouraging."

V.G.W. – "I really like Dr. Tirrito's upfront approach regarding health and exercise. It's an excellent wake-up call."

A.C. – "Ancestors on both sides of my family have had heart problems. To avoid this in myself, I became a patient of Dr. Tirrito's. Using his wellness program and with encouragement from him, I've not only lost the weight I wanted to lose, but stress tests have shown my heart and cardiovascular system to be healthier than they have ever been."

J.K. – "There are two reasons I lost 40 pounds in six months – I was determined to lose the weight and Dr. Tirrito guided me along the way."

A.F. – "I am very grateful for Dr. Tirrito and his weight management program. Since the beginning the program I have lost 50 pounds and feel great! Dr. Tirrito's program is the complete package. It continues to keep me motivated. I now have higher self-esteem, a lot of my aches and pains are gone, and shopping for clothes is much less of a hassle."

R.H. – "I do not call it a diet plan. It is a lifestyle change that I will be doing for the rest of my life. Healthy eating and regular exercise are a must to lose weight, keep the calories off, and more importantly, make you cardio healthy. As I said, this is not a diet, but a permanent way of living in order to maintain my weight. I do not hesitate to recommend this program to anyone."

So You're Fat.
Now What?

So You're Fat.
Now What?

Salvatore J. Tirrito, MD, FACC

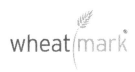

Published by Wheatmark®
610 East Delano Street, Suite 104
Tucson, Arizona 85705 U.S.A.
www.wheatmark.com

International Standard Book Number: 978-1-60494-248-4
Library of Congress Control Number: 2009921868

To my mother: Thank you for instilling in me a strong sense of intellect and desire to pursue my dreams.

To my wife: Thank you for the patience and love you have always shown me while I have pursued many endeavors.

To all my patients: Thank you for the countless hours of dialogue that we have shared, which gave me the inspiration to write this book.

TABLE OF CONTENTS

FOREWORD
....

By Dr. Troy Tompkins

AS A FAMILY PHYSICIAN, obesity and being overweight is one of the biggest causes of health issues in my practice and throughout the country. Much of the counseling I do with patients has to do with helping them lose weight. Almost all of my overweight patients want to lose weight, but the problem is finding the motivation for and maintaining the weight loss. That is why I do not advocate diets for the most part, but rather helping patients make realistic and healthy lifestyle changes. There is no secret to weight loss. The body will burn its excess fat only if one is burning more calories than one is eating. Everyone's metabolism is different, so the amount of calories that one can eat and lose weight will be different from another's. However, once a person knows how many calories they burn per day, they then have a goal of how many calories per day they can eat and still lose weight. The success is not in dieting. It is in making lifestyle changes and keeping calories in a range where weight loss is not only attainable, but can be maintained lifelong.

Dr. Tirrito's HeartWise program emphasizes healthy, lifelong lifestyle changes. That is why my patients lost nearly four hundred pounds through HeartWise last year alone. It works because it empowers people to manage their own weight loss. The goal, of course, is not weight loss for weight loss' sake, but improving health, reducing the risk of heart disease, stroke, type II diabetes, and cancer—all of which are risks increased by obesity. For some, the approach, the number crunching and calorie counting involved, can be overwhelming. One approach does not fit all. But for those who start eating less calories, eating healthier, and burning excess fat through exercise, the results are remarkable. Not only do my patients feel and look better, they are healthier and have increased self confidence because it is they who have done the hard work and are seeing the results. Is it easy? No! It is one of the hardest things in life to accomplish. Changing ingrained habits is never easy, but with all hard work comes great results. Great results are what HeartWise is all about.

— Troy Tompkins, MD

INTRODUCTION

....

SO YOU'RE FAT. NOW what? Well, join the club. An estimated ninety-seven million adults in the United States are fat. Although the primary concern about being fat for most people is their appearance, the fact is that it is a very serious health problem. Being fat substantially raises your risk of developing high blood pressure, diabetes, high cholesterol, coronary artery disease, stroke, gallbladder disease, osteoarthritis, sleep apnea, and respiratory problems, as well as endometrial, breast, prostate, and colon cancers. Being fat is the second leading cause of preventable death in the United States.

I know what you are thinking. "Oh, no! Not another diet book. What can this doctor possibly tell me that I have not already read about in another diet book?"

If you think the answer is nothing, you are exactly right.

"If you're going to tell me nothing new, then why should I read your book?" you may ask.

The answer to this question is simple: because if you read my book and follow my advice, you will lose weight and keep it off. That's a guarantee. More importantly, you will be on your way to a healthier, happier life.

Now you may be thinking to yourself, "The nerve of this guy, with all the diet books out there, to think that his book holds the secret to dieting success."

Well it does, and I won't keep you in suspense; I will tell you right here and now why this book will work for you. The truth is simple. The secret to dieting success is: *there is no secret.*

There Is No Secret

Fiction: There is some magic combination of foods that will make you lose weight. All you need are the correct proportions of carbohydrates, fats, and proteins.

Fact: If you believe this, you are only fooling yourself. Food is food. One gram of carbohydrate has approximately 4 calories. So, whether you are eating 60 grams of carbohydrates in a bowl of wheat pasta or getting those 60 grams of carbohydrates by eating a greasy plate of French fries, the equation will always be the same: 60 grams x 4 calories = 240 calories.

"Wait a minute here," you say. "Are you telling me that a plate of French fries has the same amount of calories as a bowl of wheat pasta?" No, not exactly. What I am telling you is that both have the same amount of carbohydrates. Don't forget that those poor potatoes are taken from their natural form and subjected to an oil Jacuzzi before they make their way to the table. In that Jacuzzi, those helpless potatoes are coated with oil or fat, which has a whopping 9 calories per gram. So multiply 9 calories by 30 grams (about the amount of oil that it takes to coat your potatoes), then add that 270 calories to your 240 calories worth of potatoes, and now you have a 510-calorie meal.

Is there a point to this? Yes: calories are calories. Too many diets today will lead you to believe if you eat this with that, you can eat as much as you want. Or they tell you it is okay to eat as much as you want of this, but not of that. As you read some of these books, you can almost believe that if you can find the right combination of foods, they will somehow neutralize each another when they are all mixed up in your stomach and become zero calories. That is the latest trend of diet books. They tell you, "It's what you eat and how you eat it that counts." Unfortunately, this is not true, and this is the reason why these diets ultimately fail.

So, forget about what to eat and how to eat it, and just focus on how much you eat, and you are halfway there.

You may be saying, "Wait a minute. I have a friend who was on the

South Beach Diet and lost thirty pounds. You just told me diets don't work."

Not really. I bet you that you can pick up just about any diet book out there, and if you follow its plan to the letter, you will lose some weight (at least initially). Diets do work. The South Beach Diet is the perfect example of that, and we will talk more about it later. Just do not be fooled into thinking that it is what you are eating that makes it successful. It is how much of those foods you are eating that counts. Weight Watchers, the South Beach Diet, the Sonoma Diet, etc. are successful not because they tell you what to eat, but because they tell you how much of it to eat.

Ironically, the fact that diet books sell so well is the greatest testament to the fact that they don't work (or at least don't work for long). I mean, think about it; if any of these books had the magic solution to weight loss, why would more and more diet books come out every year? In fact, why would I be writing this book at all? It is because diets don't work. People are fat and they don't want to be fat anymore. So as long as people are fat, the diet books promising the secret to long-lasting weight loss will keep rolling off the presses and make the bestseller's list every time.

"Wait! You're confusing me now. Diets are good?"

The answer is yes and no. Yes, because the South Beach and Weight Watchers diets will help you lose weight. Once again, not because they are telling you what to eat, but because they tell you how much to eat. But also no, because like every diet, the weight loss is temporary, and when you go off the diet, the pounds you shed (and usually even more) come rolling back with a vengeance.

So, should you stay on the South Beach Diet forever?

Ideally, if you could, it wouldn't be a bad idea, but human beings are not like dogs; they need a little more variety in their food choices (although I suspect dogs probably get sick and tired of eating the same food every day too). If you are some sort of human robot devoid of taste buds, you might be able to stick with whatever the diet de jour is for the rest of your life, but for the rest of us, a diet is a temporary state. When that state is over, so are your days of proudly strutting your stuff in your swimsuit.

Let's Review the Facts

Diets work, but not for the reasons you are led to believe. They work because they force you, through various methods (like point systems, meal plans, prepackaged meals, etc.), to limit the amount of calories you take in and to become more aware of how much you are eating. When you eat less, you lose weight.

Diets eventually fail because a diet is a temporary state, and when that state is over and you no longer pay attention to how much you are eating, and no longer limit your caloric intake, you eat more and you gain weight.

In this book, I'm going to show you how to take off that excess weight and keep it off.

Are you ready to change your life?

If your answer is yes, then let's get started.

ONE

....

Don't Be Afraid to Say the "F" Word

THE FIRST STEP TO a skinnier, healthier, happier you is one of self-realization. Let's face facts. You're reading a diet book; it is probably not the first one you have ever read either. You're fat! Most of us are not very comfortable using the F word, especially when we are talking about ourselves, but since you are reading this book, I think it is safe to say that you don't want to be fat anymore. Realizing that you are fat and understanding that it is not anyone else's fault but your own is a very important step to creating a new you.

We live in a society where most people have a hard time taking responsibility for the choices they make and the consequences of those choices. They would rather shift the blame for their negative experiences onto the world around them.

Are you guilty of using any of these excuses to avoid taking responsibility for being overweight?

"I am fat because there are too many fast-food restaurants."
"I am fat because my job stresses me out."
"I am fat because my spouse always has junk in the house."
"I am fat because I don't have time to exercise."
"I am fat because my kids keep me too busy."
"I am fat because my parents are fat."
"I am fat because I'm over forty."
"I'm fat because I'm big boned."
"I'm fat because I have a slow metabolism."

The excuses go and on. Taking responsibility for being fat and shifting the blame back to yourself for letting yourself get that way will ultimately make your job of losing weight easier because it is much easier to change your own behavior than to change that of the world around you.

If you truly want to lose weight and change your health and your life, just say to yourself, "I am fat. It's my fault, but I have the power to change."

You *do* have the power to change, and with my guidance, you'll lose that excess weight and this time you'll keep it off.

"So why should I care?" you ask. "I am fat, but I am okay with that." Well, first of all, if that were the case, I don't think you would be reading this book. But more importantly, let me tell you about a patient of mine; we will call her "Tina."

Meet Tina

Tina is a fifty-five-year-old woman who was sent to me by a local primary care doctor for some borderline high blood pressure, borderline high cholesterol, and borderline high blood sugars. Tina didn't really have any complaints. As far as she was concerned, she was fine. I told Tina that she could really stand to lose about thirty pounds. She became a bit angry and told me, "I know I'm fat. So what's wrong with that? I feel great. I like the way I look in the mirror. My husband loves me. My kids love me. I have lots of friends who like me for who I am. What does it matter if I'm fat?"

Realizing that I had offended Tina, I quickly tried to calm the situation. I asked Tina, "Do you use street drugs?"

She practically screamed back at me, "No! Do I look like someone who uses drugs?"

I answered, "Actually, you don't, but what is wrong with using drugs anyway?"

At this point, I suspect Tina was beginning to think that I was crazy.

She replied, "They are bad for your health. You're a doctor. You should know that."

I answered, "You're right. They're bad for your health. Now, if I could show you that being overweight was just as bad for your health, would you still be happy being overweight?"

Tina answered, "I don't see how you can compare the two. They're not the same thing."

I answered, "No, they're not. Drug use has a much more noticeable impact on a person's health and can kill you relatively quickly. Obesity has a much more subtle impact on your health and kills you slowly. However, both are killers."

Tina's interest piqued now, she asked with a half-smile, "How is being fat going to kill me?"

"What are the top two causes of death in this country?" I asked her.

"Heart attacks and strokes."

"Very good," I said. "Now, what risk factors increase your chances of having a heart attack or a stroke?"

"High blood pressure and high cholesterol."

"Right again," I said. "But you also forgot diabetes and smoking. So smoking, high blood pressure, high cholesterol, and diabetes increase your chance of having a heart attack and stroke. You don't smoke, which is great, but you do have borderline high blood pressure, borderline high cholesterol, and borderline high blood sugar. So what is the next question that I'm going to ask you?"

Tina, now understanding my line of reasoning, said, "You're going to ask me what causes high blood pressure, high cholesterol, and high blood sugars. And I'm guessing the answer is being overweight."

"Exactly," I answered. "So being overweight will kill you. It just does it in a more subtle way."

"Can't you just give me some pills to take to lower my blood pressure, cholesterol, and blood sugars?" Tina asked.

"I could, but that wouldn't be the right thing to do. First of all, your blood pressure, cholesterol, and blood sugars are only slightly elevated, not yet requiring medication. Second, do you really want to take a bunch of pills every day for the rest of your life?"

"So what should I do?" Tina asked, already knowing the answer.

We spent the next thirty minutes talking about diet and exercise. Before Tina left, I made her promise that she would at least try her best to do the things we discussed, and I told her I wanted to see her back in nine months.

Nine months later, I walked into one of my exam rooms and there was

Tina, twenty-five pounds lighter, with a smile and an unbelievable twinkle in her eyes. She gave me a big hug and spent the next fifteen minutes telling me how much her life had changed in the last nine months. She said that although she never really felt bad when she was heavier, she now realized that she also had never really felt good either. She gave me example after example of all the changes she had seen. She felt more energetic, both mentally and physically. She spent more time doing things on weekends with her kids, like bike riding. Even her sex life with her husband had gotten more passionate. In addition, if all that was not reward enough, on repeat testing, she no longer had borderline high blood pressure, cholesterol or blood sugars.

As a doctor, I see people like Tina every day, both inside and outside of the office. These are people who are fat and don't necessarily feel bad, but they also don't know how good they can feel. Here is your chance to make a change—not one that will last a week, a month, or a year, but a change that will last for the rest of your life.

The time is now, and I'm here to help you every step of the way. Throughout this book, you'll find tools to help you succeed.

Ready?

Let's go! Let's get healthy!

… And congratulations! You've just made the best decision of your life, for your life.

Two
....

How Fat Am I?

WHEN I SEE PATIENTS in the office, one of the things I comment on in my physical exam is their body mass index (BMI). For those of you not familiar with the term, body mass index is a number that is derived from your weight and your height. The real formula is:

$$\text{BMI} = \frac{\text{Weight in kilograms}}{\text{Height in meters x height in meters}}$$

This is way too complicated for most of us who never really liked the metric system. For a more familiar version of the formula, multiply your weight in pounds by the number .703. Then multiply your height in inches times your height in inches. Now divide the first number by the second number.

$$\text{BMI} = \frac{\text{Weight in pounds x .703}}{\text{Height in inches x height in inches}}$$

Example: If you are 5 feet 3 inches tall (63 inches tall) and you weigh 170 pounds, multiply 170 (your weight) x .703. This equals 119.51.

Then multiply your height in inches (63) x your height in inches (63). That equals 3,969.

Now take your first number, 119.51, and divide it by your second number, 3969. You get 30.1108. Round this number off and you have a BMI of 30 (119.510 ÷ 3,969 = 30.1108).

In my office, I actually have a table with weight on the y-axis and height (in feet and inches) on the x-axis. I quickly use it to calculate a patient's BMI.

What I want you to do now is to calculate your own BMI using the above formula. (If you are mathematically challenged, use the table in the back of the book and look up your BMI.)

Your BMI = _____

So, what is the importance of calculating your BMI? Let us first answer another question: How much do you think you should weigh? Five pounds less? Ten pounds less? Twenty pounds less? What are you basing this on?

The point of this next step is not to beat you up and make you feel bad about yourself, but to help you come up with some concrete goals in order to help you lose weight. Fat should not be defined as just how you feel. It needs to be more objective than that, because how people feel about themselves is an individual thing.

I have seen many young women in my practice who feel fat, but who are actually anorexic. If you have ever known anyone who suffers from anorexia, it is amazing to see how this disease can distort an individual's self-image.

On the other hand, I have had patients who were at the extremes of obesity and thought they were at their ideal weight. The subjective feeling of being fat varies from person to person.

To give you an example: you are reading this book, so I am going to assume you feel fat. What would it take for you to not feel fat? Losing ten pounds, twenty pounds, or thirty pounds? Being able to fit into your favorite pair of jeans, which you haven't been able to wear in years? When people start telling you, "Wow, you look like you lost weight"? Is it getting down to the weight you were at in college? Is it just feeling slimmer?

Basing your attempt to lose weight and keep it off on these very subjective feelings will ultimately lead to failure, because how you feel about yourself will change hour-to-hour and day-to-day depending upon your interactions with the world around you. You need to come up with a more objective way to decide how fat you are and how much weight you need to lose.

That is why we will use your BMI as an objective goal in losing weight. No matter how tall, short, thick, small boned or big boned you are, your BMI goal will stay the same.

You and Your BMI

A normal BMI score is 19 to 24.9, overweight is 25 to 29.9, obese is 30 to 40, and greater than 40 is morbidly obese. Is it possible to have a normal BMI and still be fat? Of course it is.

Let Me Give You an Example

Let's say you are five feet five inches tall. In order to have a BMI of 20, you would need to weigh 120 pounds, but if your BMI was 24.9, you would weigh 150 pounds. So you can have a thirty-pound increase in weight and still have a "normal" BMI. The reason is that the formula was not meant to help people lose weight; it was made to show you the risks associated with disease at various BMI levels.

People in the normal BMI range (19 to 24.9.) have no increased risk of developing health problems.

People in the overweight category (BMI 25 to 29.9) have a slightly increased risk of developing health problems (mainly high blood pressure, stroke, diabetes, heart disease, and cancer).

Those in the obese category (BMI 30 to 40) have a significantly increased risk of developing health problems.

Finally, those in the morbidly obese category (BMI greater than 40) have a serious chance of developing health problems, and in many cases their weight will dramatically shorten their lifespan.

So let's forget about pounds and how fat you think you are and keep things simple.

If your BMI is greater than 25, your goal is to get your BMI to less than 25.

If you are already less than 25 and you still feel you are fat, then try to lose enough weight to get your BMI toward the lower end of the normal range (for instance, 23, 22, or 21).

But remember, the magic number is 25. Get your BMI to less than 25, and at least then you will be at a healthy weight, and you will lower your risk of developing many serious health problems.

THREE

....

Why Am I Fat?

THE ANSWER TO THIS question is so easy and obvious that many people do not get it. *You are fat because you eat too much.*

I am sorry to break it to you this way, but for 99 percent of you fatties out there, it is not your thyroid. It is not glandular. It is not because you have a slow metabolism. It is simply because you eat too much.

Are there subtle differences in peoples' metabolisms? Yes. Is metabolism to blame for your being too fat? No.

Are there subtle genetic differences between people? Yes. Does this mean you are destined to be fat? No.

If I offend, I apologize, but the only way to be successful is to realize the truth and stop making excuses. If you accept the fact that you are fat because you are taking in more calories than you are burning up, then the solution becomes clear: burn up more calories than you take in. That is what this book is here to teach you.

Forget trying to remember:

- Which is better, wheat bread or rice?
- Which types of nuts are on my "safe" list?
- What am I not supposed to eat after dinner?
- Am I not supposed to eat fruit this week, or was that only last week?

Forget all these questions, because they will just distract you from achieving a healthier, lighter you.

Keep it simple: Eat less and burn more. That's it. Nothing else to remember.

Knowing and accepting this will be crucial in your journey to a new, leaner, healthier body. Now I want you to really think about this question for a minute: when was the last time you were at a healthy body weight (BMI <25, using the above formula)?

Or, if your BMI is less than 25 already, when was the last time you felt you were at your ideal weight?

Chances are if you really think about it, it was a long, long time ago— five, ten, maybe fifteen years ago. This brings up an important point. You didn't get fat overnight, so don't expect to get unfat overnight. Gaining weight is a gradual process and so is losing weight (if you want to keep it off).

Any diet or pill that promises you a new body in six weeks is just playing on most people's impulsiveness and impatience and conning you into wasting your money.

I know a lot of people just woke up one day, looked into the mirror, and said, "Oh my, I'm fat." And although you might feel this way, the truth is that it has been happening slowly over time. You just chose to ignore it. Getting fat in the United States of America is easy to do.

To give you an example: If you eat an extra 100 calories per day (such as you might find in a snack-sized bag of Baked Lay's potato chips or a can of soda), you will gain almost one full pound every month, or about ten pounds a year.

Let's Take a Closer Look

John is five-foot-ten, forty-four years old, and living in beautiful Tucson, Arizona. When he was in college, he played several varsity sports and was in the best shape of his life (155 pounds, BMI at 22).

After graduating from college (at age twenty-four) and becoming a financial analyst, he now spends most of his time driving around town meeting with clients. He is always on the go, so he eats most of his meals in his car—meals he picks up from the closest fast-food restaurant.

He gets home around 7 PM, and on his way home, he usually picks up Chinese food or pizza for him and his wife (age forty), and their three kids (ages ten, twelve, and fifteen).

After dinner, he spends a little time with his wife and kids, and then he and his wife go to bed. He then does the same thing the next day. He loves his weekends and always has some grand plan (like going hiking or going for a ride on his new bike, which has been sitting in the garage collecting dust), but his plans never seem to work out the way he wants. He has to run errands with his wife, participates in activities with his kids, or is just too tired and burned out from the workweek to even think about moving off the couch.

Let's give John the benefit of the doubt and say that since leaving college he has gained only about four pounds per year (about a third of a pound per month). Now at age forty-four, John weighs an impressive 235 pounds. His BMI is almost 33.

He has a forty-four-inch waist, has to lean all the way forward to see his toes, and gets wiped out walking up a flight of steps (which he vehemently avoids), or carrying groceries in from the car. He looks at himself, he looks at his wife (who is about thirty pounds heavier than when they got married), and he looks at his kids (who spend most of their free time playing video games and eating junk food), and thinks to himself, "Where did I go wrong?"

This little scenario unfortunately correctly describes the bulk of Americans: overweight and sedentary, with poor eating habits.

Perhaps, the greatest crime is not that John and his wife let themselves go, but the example they are setting for their children. Their lifestyle is telling their children that it is okay to be fat and sedentary. Their three kids will grow up to be fat and have fat families of their own. How can you expect anything else when it is all they know?

There are many other reasons that people put on weight, like becoming inactive after an injury or illness, quitting smoking, being under a lot of stress, going through menopause, etc. However, except for the very rare hormonal imbalance, the reason for weight gain is still the same: you have violated the immutable law of weight loss.

The immutable law of weight loss is, "Don't eat more calories than you burn off."

So, as we said above, regardless of your reason for getting fat, the answer is still the same:

Eat less and burn more.

Four

......

Getting Started

BEFORE WE CAN GET started on the road to weight loss, we must remind ourselves how we got here in the first place: by eating too much. So, the next logical question you have to ask yourself is, "How much should I eat in a day?"

The way we are going to figure that out is by calculating your *basal metabolic rate* (BMR).

BMR Formula:

Women:	BMR = 655 + (4.35 x weight in pounds) + (4.7 x height in inches) – (4.7 x age in years)
Men:	BMR = 66 + (6.23 x weight in pounds) + (12.7 x height in inches) – (6.8 x age in years)

Your BMR _____

So what does this number mean?

Basal metabolic rate is the amount of energy (measured in calories) required to keep your body functioning every day, assuming that you are completely inactive. This includes processes like the beating of your heart, breathing, and maintaining body temperature.

What are some of the things that we can learn from the above formula?

First, the taller you are and the heavier you are, the higher your metabolic rate will be. This is just basic physics. It takes energy to move any object, and the bigger its mass, the more energy it takes to move it.

Also, notice in the formula that age is subtracted from all the other variables, telling us that the older we are, the lower our BMR will be. This is not rocket science. Just about anyone can attest to the fact that as you mature, you just can't eat the way you used to when you were twenty. The reason is that younger people have faster metabolisms. This is because there are more active processes going on (i.e., growing) inside their bodies.

Don't get discouraged. You can still lose weight as you get older. It will just come off a little slower than when you were younger.

What We Can Learn From Jane and Barbara: An Example:

Take Jane, a forty-year-old woman who is five-five and weighs 170 pounds (BMI = 28). Using the above formula for women, her BMR would be 1512 calories per day: $(655 + (4.35 \times 170) + (4.7 \times 65)) - 4.7 \times 40$. In other words, if Jane just sat in a chair for twenty-four hours, she would burn up roughly 1500 calories.

Now let us look at Barbara, who is also forty years old and five-foot-five, but she weighs 250 pounds (BMI = 41.6). Her BMR would be 1859 calories per day: $655 + (4.35 \times 250) + (4.7 \times 65) - (4.7 \times 40)$.

If both Jane and Barbara go on the South Beach Diet and eat a calorie-restricted diet (which is all the South Beach Diet is) of 1300 calories per day, who will lose more weight? Barbara does, of course.

Why? Because, assuming all other factors are equal, Barbara is negative approximately 550 calories per day, while Jane is negative only about 200 calories per day. Since a pound of fat is approximately 3500 calories, it will take Barbara about six days to lose one pound of fat and Jane about eighteen days to lose the same amount. Or, for every pound of fat Jane loses, Barbara will lose three pounds.

To simplify, here's how Jane and Barbara's BMRs minus their 1300-per-day caloric intake would look:

Jane's BMR is	=	1512
Jane's caloric intake	=	1300 calories per day
Jane will be negative		212 calories per day
Barbara's BMR is	=	1859
Barbara caloric intake	=	1300 calories per day
Barbara will be negative		559 calories per day

So again, if Jane and Barbara do nothing but sit in a chair for six months and eat their South Beach, 1300-calorie-per-day diet, Barbara will lose thirty pounds and Jane will lose only ten pounds.

Let's say after six months, Jane (now 160 pounds, with a BMI of 27) gets discouraged after only losing ten pounds and quits, but Barbara (now 220 pounds, with a BMI of 37) is tickled with her progress and wants to lose more. So she does the same thing she has been doing, but notices the weight does not seem to be coming off like it had over the last six months. That is because Barbara is not the same woman she was six months ago (literally). At 220 pounds, her BMR has dropped to approximately 1700 calories. So, on the same 1300-calorie-per-day diet, she is negative only 400 calories each day.

Remembering that a pound of fat is about 3500 calories, it now takes Barbara nine days to lose the same pound of fat that had initially taken only six days (when she weighed 250 pounds). Since she has not had the benefit of reading my book (and doesn't understand how her weight affects her BMR), all she sees is her weight loss slowing down or stopping, and she gets discouraged and quits. This illustrates an important point. *Real weight loss takes a long time.* Think about how long it took you to get as heavy as you are. It took a while to pack on an extra thirty pounds, and it will take at least as long (and usually longer) to lose it.

What do I mean by *real weight loss*? Real weight loss means losing fat. Be very wary of any diet that promises you quick results. When a diet makes you ten pounds slimmer in ten days, I promise you it is not ten pounds of fat you are losing. What you are losing is mostly water, a couple pounds of partially digested food in your colon, a few pounds of muscle, and virtually no fat.

Your body is about 60 percent water, so you can actually lose a fair amount of weight quickly if you dehydrate yourself, which is what many of these rapid-weight-loss diets do. The problem is that it is only a temporary state; as soon as you go off the diet and start eating and drinking again, the weight comes right back. More importantly, it is extremely unhealthy.

Your body is 60 percent water for a reason; it needs it to perform vital everyday functions. So, give up the idea of the quick permanent-weight-loss solution. It is a myth.

Real weight loss takes time. Realize it, accept it, be patient, and you will ultimately succeed.

Can I Change My BMR?

Can you change your basal metabolic rate? The good news is you can, at least a little. Your BMR is influenced not only by your age, weight, height, and gender, but also by a multitude of other factors, such as environmental temperature, dieting, and exercise habits.

Muscle is more metabolically active than fat. Look at your arm and contract your bicep. What happens? It changes shape. That is because thousands of muscle fibers attach to thousands of other muscle fibers to cause the muscle to contract. This takes energy, which means *burning calories.*

Now, look at some fat; your abdomen is usually a good place. Smack it and see what happens. It jiggles. Now that jiggle, although it might be entertaining, is a passive process not requiring much energy (i.e., burning many calories). Because men tend to have more muscle, they generally have a higher BMR than women—remember the above formula.

People living in the extremes of temperature (really cold or hot climates) generally have higher BMRs than those living in more temperate climates. This is because sweating and shivering burns calories.

In general, depending on the intensity and duration, consistent exercise will also increase your BMR. We will talk a lot about this later.

Also, certain diets can dramatically affect your BMR (unfortunately, in a very negative way), so this seems like a perfect time to mention a thing or two about starvation diets.

Insider's Tip: Why Starvation Diets Don't Work

Before I get to the next section, I would like to spend a few minutes talking about a diet plan that has stood the test of time ... as being the most ridiculous, unsuccessful, and dangerous way to try to lose weight. The starvation diet is still out there in various forms and it still does not work.

The theory of the starvation diet is pretty simple. If you eat practically nothing, you will lose weight. Unfortunately (or fortunately, depending on how you look at it), the human body is a little too smart.

An Example

Let's use Jane (five-foot-five and 170 pounds) from the above example. We've established that assuming she does nothing, she will burn up about 1500 calories per day. Let's say she is desperate. Her twenty-year high school reunion is coming up and she wants to look good. She didn't get the results she was hoping for on the South Beach Diet, eating 1300 calories per day, so she takes things up a notch. Jane decides that she is going to eat only 800 calories a day.

According to what we have just learned, this means that Jane will be negative 700 calories (1500 minus 800) per day. A pound of fat is 3500 calories, so Jane should lose about a pound every five days. In six months, she should be down about thirty-six pounds—at a weight of 134 —looking trim and slim, right? Well, initially she will lose a little more than one pound every five days, because if you stop eating (which is essentially what eating 800 calories per day is like), you are likely to drop a little extra weight after going to the bathroom a few times and getting rid of what was hanging around in your colon.

So, let's say five days go by and Jane loses four pounds. She's now 166 pounds. She is happy with what she sees on the scale and, although she's hungry every second that she is awake, she is determined to stick it out.

Another five days go by and Jane loses another two pounds. She now weighs 164. She is not as happy, but is still determined. Another five days, and she loses another pound (163 pounds). Jane is a bit discouraged, but unwilling to give up. Five more days, and this time when she jumps on the scale she finds it has not changed. She is still 163 pounds!

Now, not only is Jane hungry, but angry—a very dangerous combination. Even worse, she looks up from bathroom scale, looks in the mirror, and is horrified by what she sees. She has big dark circles under eyes and her skin is paper thin. She has blemishes all over her face. Her gums are swollen and bleeding. Her nails are brittle and cracked. Her hair no longer has that natural shine; it seems dull and course. She runs her hand through it and she is aghast as clumps of it come out in her hand. Jane turns from that mirror and runs out of the room. Thinking she is dying of some horrible disease, she calls her doctor to schedule an appointment.

If Jane showed up in my office, I would like to think that the diagnosis would be apparent. But even if I didn't get it right away, I am sure it would be clear once Jane opened her mouth, because there is nothing more revealing than the stench of death on someone's breath when they are starving to death and malnourished. That stench, which really does smell like decaying flesh, is telltale. I have diagnosed many people with eating disorders that way. It really is your body decaying, or at least starting to break down, in order to sustain life.

Your body is smarter than you think, and it doesn't want to die. So, when it faces a situation where it thinks it could (like when it only gets 800 calories a day), it adapts. It starts shutting down nonessential but important processes, like making nutrients to keep your hair and nails strong, and making oils to protect your skin. It also starts breaking down muscle in order to use that protein for other vital processes. Essentially, your body goes into hibernation mode and only performs the functions absolutely necessary to live.

As week after week goes by at 800 calories per day, more and more body processes slow and shut down. As more and more processes shut down, and your body needs less energy, your BMR slowly begins to drop. 1200 calories per day … 1000 calories per day … 900 calories per day … After a few weeks, your BMR will match the amount of calories coming in, and you stop losing weight.

So, Jane sees her doctor. He correctly arrives at the diagnosis and tells her she is not dying, she is just malnourished. Relieved that she is not dying, she heads over to McDonald's and starts eating. She takes her first huge bite of a Big Mac and, although it tastes good, as soon as it hits her stomach, she doesn't feel very well. Her stomach is cramping up and she feels sick and fights the urge to vomit. Why? Because her body has been running on backup power and has turned off many of the processes necessary to digest that big bolus of food. Also, her stomach has shrunk considerably.

Jane waits, and the feeling eventually passes. She decides to eat a little more slowly. She goes back to her old eating habits, about 1500 calories per day, and two days later she is up four pounds. Her weight now is 167. Two days later, she's up three more pounds, back to 170, and one week after that, she is 175 pounds. So, roughly, one month after beginning her starvation diet, Jane is five pounds heavier and is just starting to get that shine back in her hair and that luster back in her skin.

Well, I said the body is smart, but it's not that smart. It doesn't realize that the starvation it has had to endure over the last few weeks is intentional. Your body isn't taking any chances, so in addition to repairing the damage done, it stores as many calories as it can as fat, just in case. That means you really pack on the pounds.

Also remember that over the last few weeks of starvation, the BMR drops in an attempt to limit that calorie deficit. It takes a while for the BMR to return to normal. So if Jane starts eating 1500 calories per day again and her BMR is only 600 calories per day, she is going to be positive 900 calories per day, which will quickly add up to pounds.

Fortunately, your body has a relatively short memory, and after a few weeks of eating normally, your BMR will come back to its original level and you will be back to where you started—actually, five pounds heavier.

I hope this has been an informative, yet somewhat graphic demonstration of why starvation diets don't work. So what is the answer?

Proper nutrition and exercise!

FIVE

Calculating Your Intake: Nutrition 101

IN THIS CHAPTER WE are going to start building an understanding of basic nutrition and go over a few basic terms. We will then use this knowledge to construct a meal plan that obeys the three rules of weight loss, which we will discuss below.

All food is essentially composed of three elements: carbohydrates, proteins, and fats.

Carbohydrates

Carbohydrates come from a wide array of foods. Some examples are bread, rice, beans, milk, juice, popcorn, chips, potatoes, cookies, spaghetti, corn, and candy. They also come in a variety of forms. The most common and abundant are sugars, fibers, and starches.

The basic building block of a carbohydrate is a sugar molecule like glucose, fructose, or sucrose. These are also known as simple sugars.

When a bunch of sugar molecules are linked together in various configurations, sometimes containing hundreds of individual sugar molecules, they are called complex carbohydrates. Complex carbohydrates are your starches and fibers.

The digestive system handles all carbohydrates, whether simple sugars or complex carbohydrates, in the same way. Since all carbohydrates' basic building blocks are simple sugars, the digestive system, through an array of enzymes, tries to break them down and turn them back to their original form. Once back in the form of simple sugars, your body converts most of the other simple sugars (fructose and sucrose) into glucose, because cells are designed to use this as a universal energy source.

Fiber is an exception to this rule. Fiber is a complex array of linked sugar molecules, which your body does not possess the right enzymes to digest. Since it can't be broken down into individual sugar molecules and absorbed by the digestive system, it passes through the body undigested. Fiber is an important part of your diet because, for lack of a better term, it keeps you "regular." It helps keep things moving in your colon by grabbing undigested food and toxins on its way through. Think of fiber as a little snowball sitting on top of a big mountain. If you take that snowball and roll it down the mountain, it will pick up more snow and whatever else is in its path on its way down, and by the time it gets to the bottom, it is a lot bigger than when it started. That is kind of like what happens in your colon when you eat foods high in fiber.

For a more complete list of foods containing carbohydrates, see the back of the book.

Hot Topic: Carbohydrates and the Glycemic Index

A new concept, which has taken the dieting world by storm, is known as the *glycemic index.* It measures how fast and how far blood sugar rises after you eat a food that contains carbohydrates. Foods like white bread and white rice are converted very quickly to glucose and are classified as having a high glycemic index. Brown rice or wheat bread, in contrast, are converted more slowly to glucose and have a low glycemic index. Why is this important and why has it become a popular selling point for a lot of diet books?

When glucose enters the bloodstream, your body makes insulin. Your body's goal is to get that glucose out of your bloodstream and into your cells, where it can be used immediately to make energy or stored for use at a later time. The higher your blood glucose level, the more insulin your body makes—to the point where it makes too much and eventually causes your blood sugar level to drop.

As we will discuss below, when your blood sugar drops too low you get hungry. Since foods with a high glycemic index are converted to glucose and are absorbed more quickly, they tend to raise your blood sugar higher, which, through the action of insulin, eventually causes your blood sugar to drop too low, making you hungry.

Foods with a low glycemic index, since they are converted to glucose and absorbed more slowly, don't cause the oversecretion of insulin that leads to low blood sugars.

So there is nothing wrong with white bread. Calories are calories, and white and wheat bread have pretty much the same amount. The reason most diet books try to steer you away from white bread and other foods with a high glycemic index is to keep you from getting too hungry.

For a list of the glycemic indices of various foods, see the back of the book.

Proteins

Take away the water, and about 75 percent of your weight is protein. Protein is in muscle, bone, skin, hair, and virtually every other body part or tissue. It makes up the enzymes that power thousands of chemical reactions that allow you to do things like see, think, breathe, and eat. At least ten thousand different proteins make you what you are and keep you that way.

Protein in food is digested and broken down into its most basic form, amino acids. Once these amino acids are absorbed, the body uses them to build new proteins to replace and repair the ones already there. Because the body doesn't store amino acids as it does fats or carbohydrates, it needs a daily supply to keep the body functioning normally. Proteins, unlike fats and carbohydrates, are not very efficient sources of energy. However, in an emergency, your body will start breaking down proteins to use as energy (remember the starvation diet above).

So, what foods contain protein? Just think of yourself. Animals and anything that comes from an animal (like milk, cheese, and eggs) has protein. Luckily, especially if you are a vegetarian, there are also many nonanimal sources of protein. Foods like nuts, beans, and other legumes are good sources of protein. For a more complete list of foods containing protein, refer to the back of the book.

Fats

For as long as diets have been around, people have viewed the word "fat" in a negative way. When you say to someone, "You are fat," you are not complimenting him or her. So, how did one of the three basic elements of food become a way to describe someone's physical appearance? Instead of saying "You are fat," why don't we say, "You are carbohydrate," or "You are protein"?

The reason has to do with many of the properties of fats. Fats are essential for the human body to function, but it needs them in very small amounts. As we learned above, one gram of fat has twice the amount of calories as one gram of carbohydrates or protein. So from an evolutionary point of view, it makes perfect sense that our bodies would choose to store fat instead of protein or carbohydrates as a long-term energy source.

Remember, your body's job is not to look pretty; its job is to stay alive, and back in the days when food was not so easy to come by, it stored as much energy (as fat) as it could. It is hard to change millions of years of evolution, and your body doesn't understand that the next meal is right around the corner and there is no need to store all this extra fuel. Instead, your body does what it was made to do; and day after day, month after month, year after year, you get fatter and fatter.

Fats Can Be Broken Down into Essentially Four Types:

1. Monounsaturated fats
2. Polyunsaturated fats
3. Saturated fats
4. Trans fats

Monounsaturated fat comes from sources such as:

- Olives
- Olive oil
- Canola oil
- Peanut oil
- Cashews
- Almonds
- Peanuts and most other nuts
- Avocados

Monounsaturated fat is one of the so-called good fats and can help lower your LDL (bad cholesterol) and raise your HDL (good cholesterol). We will talk more about cholesterol later.

Polyunsaturated fat comes from such sources as:

- Corn
- Soybean
- Safflower and cottonseed oils
- Fish

Polyunsaturated fat is another of the so-called good fats that can help lower LDL and raise your HDL.

Saturated fat comes from sources such as:

- Whole milk
- Butter
- Cheese
- Ice cream
- Meat
- Chocolate
- Coconuts
- Coconut milk
- Coconut oil

Saturated fat is considered one of the bad fats that raise both LDL and HDL.

Trans fats are unique because they are artificially created. Trans fats are produced when hydrogen gas reacts with oil. Many manufacturers started including trans fats in their processed foods about twenty years ago to prolong their products' shelf life. They are found in:

- Most margarine
- Vegetable shortenings
- Partially hydrogenated vegetable oils
- Deep-fried chips

- Many fast foods
- Most commercially baked goods

Trans fats are thought to be even worse than saturated fats because they not only raise your LDL, but also lower your HDL. (For a more complete list of high-fat foods, see the back of the book.) So the reason the word "fat" has such a stigma attached to it is for the two reasons mentioned above. They have twice the amount of calories as equivalent amounts of proteins or carbohydrates. In addition, saturated and trans fats contribute to coronary artery disease.

Now for the two questions I bet you are dying to ask: "Can I get fat if I don't eat any fat?" and "Will I develop coronary artery disease if I don't eat any fat?"

I will answer the first question now and answer the second question in Chapter 8.

Yes, you can get fat even if you eat no fat.

The reason this is possible is that your body will take carbohydrates, break them down, and turn them into fat, which it will then store. Your body is a lot smarter than you are and it will always find a way to do what it is supposed to do: survive.

Now that we have a better understanding of basic nutrition, here are some meal plans from two very popular diets that I have put together in the following table. I happened to choose certain days from the meal plans for comparison, but I promise you that whatever days, or meal plans, or diets you look at, you will find the same things. Let's examine the table very closely.

A Comparison of South Beach and Sonoma Diet Meal Plans

	South Beach: Phase 1, Day 1	Sonoma Diet: Phase 1, Day 1	South Beach: Phase 2, Day 1	Sonoma Diet: Phase 2, Day 1
Breakfast	6 oz vegetable juice, 2 Decaf coffee or tea with sugar substitute and nonfat milk, vegetable quiche **Calories: 254**	2 scrambled eggs, 1 slice whole grain toast **Calories: 270**	1 cup fresh strawberries, oatmeal with milk and walnuts. Decaf coffee or tea with sugar substitute and nonfat milk **Calories: 343**	Whole grain cereal and milk **Calories: 170**
Snack	1 part-skim mozzarella stick **Calories: 80**	**WOMEN ONLY** 11 almonds (split up during the day as snacks) **Calories: 77**	1 hardboiled egg **Calories: 80**	**WOMEN ONLY** 2 stalks celery with 2 Tbsp peanut butter, 22 almonds (split up during day) **Calories: 404**
Lunch	Sliced grilled chicken breast on romaine, 2 Tbsp balsamic vinaigrette, sugar-free Jell-O **Calories: 260**	Greek salad with grilled shrimp in ½ of a whole wheat pita **Calories: 369**	Mediterranean chicken salad **Calories: 220**	Tangy black bean soup, spinach salad with vinaigrette, 1 cup of berries **Calories: 475**
Snack	Celery stuffed with 1 wedge of laughing cow light cheese **Calories: 40**	**MEN ONLY** 33 almonds (split up during the day) **Calories: 231**	Fresh pear with 1 wedge of laughing cow cheese **Calories: 130**	2 mozzarella string cheese sticks, 2 celery stalks with 2 Tbsp peanut butter; **MEN ONLY:** 33 almonds (split up during the day) **Calories: 600**
Dinner	Grilled salmon with rosemary, steamed asparagus, tossed salad, olive oil, and vinegar **Calories: 348**	Chicken en papillote with vegetables **Calories: 249**	Spinach stuffed salmon fillet, vegetable medley. Tossed salad, olive and vinegar **Calories: 424**	Latin spiced pork tenderloin, toasted quinoa pilaf, roasted zucchini, ½ cup of cantaloupe **Calories: 403**
Snack	Vanilla ricotta crème **Calories: 178**		Chocolate dipped strawberries **Calories: 175**	
Total Calories	1160 (men and women)	965 (women), 1119 (men)	1372 (men and women)	1452 (women), 1648 (men)

The first thing that I want you to notice on the diet comparison chart is the total number of calories. It ranges from 965 to 1648 per day. For those of you who don't know much about calories, that is not a lot. To put things in perspective, a Big Mac, large fries, and a milkshake is 1265 calories, and that is only one meal. According to the U.S. Department of Agriculture, the average American eats about 2700 calories per day.

The next thing I want you to notice is that both the above diets have a phase 1 in which you eat fewer calories than in phase 2. Now, here is a question that should be easy for you to answer. When you start a diet, when do you lose more weight? Toward the beginning or end?

Most people who follow a diet closely tend to lose more weight in the first one to two weeks, and then the weight loss slows down. This is due to several reasons which we will talk about later, and one very important reason which we will talk about now.

You start your diet, and you go from 2700 calories per day to about 1000 calories per day (if we average Phase 1 days of the South Beach and Sonoma diets). That is 1,700 calories less per day. You will lose weight, that's for certain, but you will be pretty damn irritable, because going from 2700 to 1,000 calories will leave you feeling hungry.

This brings me to the next similarity between the two diets and all modern weight loss plans. You are always eating. Counting meals and snacks, you eat a minimum of five times per day.

Let's Look At An Example: "George"

I recently had a patient—let's call him George—lose twenty-five pounds. George, who is five-ten, was a good forty-five pounds above his ideal body weight, and had been stuck there for as long as he could remember. When I asked George how he lost the weight, he said he stopped skipping breakfast.

Now, is it possible that George lost weight by adding an extra meal to the day?

Since George was convinced that he had invented a miracle diet that would allow you to lose weight by eating more, I asked him to write down what he normally ate in an average day, before and after he started eating breakfast. After adding up all the calories, it became crystal clear to George that he was eating a lot less after adding breakfast.

What George had done before he started eating breakfast was start his day with a huge lunch, about 1000 to 1300 calories, because by the time lunch rolled around, he was starving. He would be stuffed for a while, but eventually as the evening rolled on, he would get hungry again and eat an even bigger dinner, about 1500 to 1700 calories. He also tended to eat his dinners very late, partly because he was so full from lunch, and partly because by eating late, he wasn't too hungry the next morning.

So, in only two meals, George was packing away an impressive 2500 to 3000 calories per day. Looking back, he says that he was always in one of two modes: starving or stuffed.

A lot of Americans tend to live their lives just like George and end up either stuffed or starving. For two big reasons, this not conducive to weight loss.

When George started adding in breakfast, because he wasn't a big morning eater, his meals tended to be something simple—for instance, cereal with milk, a bagel with coffee, or eggs and toast. His morning meals averaged about 250 to 300 calories. By the time lunch rolled around, he wasn't starving like he had always been in the past. Without thinking about it, he stopped overeating. His average lunch intake went down to about 400 to 600 calories..

Then, because he was eating a smaller meal at lunchtime, he ate his dinner earlier. As an added benefit, since he did not gorge himself at lunch anymore, he was not as hungry by dinnertime as he had been in the past. As a result, he had a more sensible dinner, about 500 to 700 calories.

Since he was eating dinner a little earlier, he got a little hungry toward the late evening and starting having a snack (usually a scoop of ice cream or frozen yogurt), which was about 150 to 200 calories.

George went from two meals per day to four, but his total caloric intake actually dropped to about 1250 to 1800 calories per day. If you do the math, George was eating about 1200 to 1700 fewer calories per day. Of course he lost weight!

Meals	Old George	New George
Breakfast	Skipped	250–300 calories
Lunch	1000–1300 calories	400–600 calories
Dinner	1500–1700 calories	500–700 calories
Snack	None	150–200 calories
Total	2500–3000 calories/day	1300–1800 calories/day

Now, let's see if you were really paying attention to what you just read. If you were, then you must be wondering if I really meant it when I said George was *less* hungry at dinnertime because he ate a smaller lunch.

Well I did mean it, because it is exactly right. It's called "rebound hunger." When a huge bolus of food hits your stomach (like a Big Mac and large fries), it diverts a lot of its resources to digesting and absorbing that meal. One of the primary players in this is insulin.

As mentioned previously, in very simple terms, insulin's role is to help get sugar out of your bloodstream and into your cells so that your blood sugar level does not get too high and make you sick. The bigger the meal, the more insulin your body secretes, to the point where it overcompensates and causes your blood sugar to drop too low.

What happens when your blood sugar drops? You get hungry—very hungry.

So when George cut down the size of his lunches, his body secreted less insulin, which caused less of a drop in his blood sugar, which then made him feel less hungry.

Now let us get back to examining our diet plans. The next similarities I want you to notice between the South Beach and Sonoma diets are the food choices. If you compare the meals and snacks in all of the columns, you should notice that they are pretty much the same: mostly high in lean protein, complex carbohydrates, and unsaturated fats.

If you are not a budding nutritionist, this might not be readily apparent, so please take my word for it. Let's at least agree that when you look down the columns, the foods look pretty similar.

The fact that the food choices are almost identical, believe me, is not by chance. Most popular (and successful) diets today emphasize lean protein, complex carbs, and unsaturated fat for two main reasons. First, as we learned above, it takes longer to digest protein, fats, and complex carbs, so you stay full longer. Second, by avoiding simple sugars, your insulin levels do not overcompensate and cause hypoglycemia and rebound hunger.

So remember, for a diet to work it has to do three things:

1. Get you to eat less (by making you eat more frequently).
2. Keep you satisfied (by eating foods that take longer to digest).
3. Prevent rebound hunger (by avoiding foods that will excessively lower your blood sugar).

Getting back to one of the original points that I made in the introduction, diets are not necessarily all bad. They can teach you to make good food choices that promote weight loss. However, rather than just blindly following the meal plans they give you, it is important to understand why you are eating what you are eating, because one day the diet will end and you'll want to be able to make the right choices on your own. If you walked into my office and I said, "Mr. or Ms. X, you need to take this pill," I would hope that you would ask why and not just take it. It is the same with a diet. Understand why you are doing what you are doing so you can make the right choices by yourself.

Now we are going to make healthier food choices by making a log and tracking everything we eat and drink. It will be identical to the sample table below, except that you are going to enter your own food choices.

What you need to do is learn to count calories. Use either a calorie-counting book (if you already have one), or use one of the free calorie charts that you can find on the Internet (See the back of the book for a list of websites).

You need to keep track of everything you eat and record the number of calories to get a good idea of just how many calories are going into your body each day. When you are ready to start filling in your own chart, just make photocopies of the blank caloric intake tables I have provided for you in the back of the book and start filling them in.

On the following page, I have provided you with a sample table to help get you started.

Sample Table to Track Your Caloric Intake

	Mon.	Tues.	Wed.	Thurs.	Fri.	Sat.	Sun.
Breakfast	Whole grain cereal with nonfat milk 270	2 eggs with a glass of nonfat milk and 2 links of soy links 300	McDonald's Sausage McMuffin, egg and hash-browns, 8 oz OJ 630	3 Aunt Jemima, Original Mix pancakes with ¼ cup syrup and 8 oz OJ 580	Everything bagel with garden veggie cream cheese, Coke 500	All you can eat breakfast buffet 2000	Starbucks Grande Café Vanilla Frappuccino and blueberry muffin 910
Snack	Granola bar 140	Energy bar 140	Granola parfait 220	Banana 110	4 oz bag of gummy worms 520	No snack	4 oz bag of Pepper Jack Doritos 600
Lunch	2 slices wheat bread with tuna salad (2 eggs, tuna, pickles, nonfat mayo) 620	Greek salad (from Noodles) 409	Caesar salad with Caesar dressing 317	PBJ smoothie from Planet Smoothie 560	2 slices of wheat bread and 4 oz turkey with 1 slice of nonfat cheese 410	Schlotzsky's Deli Original Sandwich, regular 16-oz Coke 975	4 oz peanut butter and 4 oz jelly sandwich, glass of whole milk 640
Snack	Thin crisps 100	Apple with peanut butter 270	No snack	Soy nuts 140	Snack mix 150	Baked Lay's Potatoes (4 oz), chips, Coke 550	2 mozzarella cheese sticks 160
Dinner	Wheat pasta with garlic and oil 450	Meatloaf (Healthy Choice) with garlic breadsticks 436	Personal pan cheese pizza (Pizza Hut) and 16-oz Coke 830	Dinner at restaurant (appetizer, soup, main course, and dessert) 2000	Grilled 4-oz swordfish with green beans 196	Thai curry beef and vegetables 443	Cheeseburger, French fries, 8-oz Sprite 857
Snack	Low-fat ice cream sandwich 150	2 graham crackers 120	Ben & Jerry's Chunky Monkey (1 pint) 1240		Medium Dairy Queen Blizzard chocolate chip cookie dough 950	No snack	Key lime pie 590
Total	1730	1675	3237	3390	2726	3968	3757
				Weekly 20,483			

I compiled this table by asking friends, family, patients, and random strangers to list what they ate for a particular meal. When I had enough meals to fill this chart, I entered them in a semi-random fashion. Let's examine the table closely.

The first thing you should notice is the wide variation in calories and meals. The food choices from Monday and Tuesday came from people I knew ate a reasonable, healthy diet; the rest of the week represented more of the "average man on the street" food choices. The caloric differences between Monday and Tuesday and the rest of the week is dramatic and clearly demonstrates why the majority of Americans are fat.

In the last chapter, you learned to calculate your BMR, so you should now have an idea of how many calories you burn in a day while at rest. Look at some of the meals above. It is easy—way too easy—to see how you can eat your entire BMR in one or two meals, or even a snack.

Insider's Tip: Dining Out

As I am sure you have already figured out from looking at the above table, eating out (whether at a sit-down or take-out restaurant) is the mortal enemy of every dieter. I will go as far to say that if you eat out more than twice a week, you are probably never going to lose any weight. The best advice I can give you is, don't eat out. However, if you have to, let me give you a few helpful rules to follow:

1. Almost every fast-food restaurant offers nutritional information about the various menu items. Ask for it. If it is not available in the restaurant, you can usually find it on the Internet. In the back of the book, I have included links to many popular fast-food restaurant websites to help you to make "relatively" healthy fast-food choices.

2. When you go out to a restaurant, you are pretty much at their mercy. With the exception of a few chains that list the number of calories for some of their meals (like Chili's, PF Chang's, and Applebee's), you are not going to be able to calculate how many calories you are eating when you dine out. Don't stress out about it and ruin your meal. Remember the chapter you read on nutrition. Try to make sensible food choices and follow these rules:

A. **Don't overeat.** Don't feel you need to finish everything on your plate.

B. **Watch the free stuff.** Whether it is bread, crackers, or a sample of an appetizer, just because it is free doesn't mean it is free of calories. Try to avoid these free temptations to cut calories from an already calorie-rich meal.

C. **Beverages** can add a significant number of calories to your meal, so watch out.

D. Rather than trying to figure out how many calories are in each course, **use the estimated values** I've provided and you'll be reasonably close.

> **Appetizer**: 600 calories;
> **Soup or salad**: 400 calories (as a side);
> **Main course**: 1000 calories;
> **Dessert**: 600 calories.

For example, Thursday night you go out to dinner and you have an appetizer and main course. You then go to your chart and find the box that corresponds to "Thursday dinner." Using the quick estimates of values above, fill in 1100 calories (appetizer 600 calories + Main Course 1000 = 1600 calories). I am being very conservative here. In today's "more is better" society it is not uncommon to go to a restaurant and find that your favorite appetizer is several thousand calories alone!!!

E. **All-you-can-eat buffets**: If you are one that truly takes advantage of the all-you-can-eat buffet, fill in 2000 calories in your caloric intake chart. (That is being generous.)

These are just guides. For some meals you will probably underestimate the amount of calories you have eaten, and for others you will likely overestimate. If you think you can do a better job yourself, bring your calorie-counter book with you, or try looking up everything you ate when you get home. Ask the chef. You might get lucky, and the chef might be able to tell you about how many calories are in the dishes he or she prepares.

Just remember though: Eating out a lot and losing weight mix about as well as oil and water. They don't go very well together. If you are serious about losing weight, eat at home.

Hot Topic: Supersized America

As I just stated, the rules of eating out are just guidelines, and guidelines tend to change. This is especially true today because we live in a country of supersized people eating supersized meals. There used to be a time when you could go into a restaurant, order a salad or an entrée, and actually be eating a relatively light meal. Not anymore.

The supersized meal appears to have originated in the fast food industry, but now it can be seen everywhere, from mom and pop restaurants to grocery stores and coffeehouses. In fact, there are very few things left that can't be supersized. So what does this all mean? Look around. You are living in a country of fat people who are eating ridiculously large meals that cause them to get even fatter, and sentencing themselves to a life of chronic disease and an early death. But if you are one of those people, don't blame the fast-food industry, as ultimately you decide what goes into your mouth. Remember, you are in control and you determine your own fate.

A Few Words About Alcohol

Just about everyone loves a nice drink every now and again, and from a health perspective there is nothing wrong with alcohol consumption in moderation. In fact, the incidence of heart disease in those who drink moderate amounts of alcohol (no more than two drinks per day for men or one drink per day for women) is lower than in nondrinkers. However, from a weight-loss perspective, alcohol is your enemy. Whether you are relaxing at home, hanging out at a friend's house, or enjoying a nice meal, you must remember that with each drink you are consuming extra calories, and those calories can add up quickly.

Let's Look at an Example

You are out at a nice restaurant with your significant other, and through the course of your 2000-calorie meal (appetizer, soup, salad, main course, and dessert), you have three vodka martinis (210 calories each) and then finish the meal off with a cup of Irish coffee (218 calories). You have added 848 calories to your 2000-calorie meal, giving you a grand total of 2848 calories. That is just one meal! Even if you ate light during the day, you still probably took in about 4000 calories for the day.

And you wonder why you can't lose weight?

Approximate Number of Calories in Some Common Alcoholic Beverages

- **Beer (12 fluid ounces):** about 100 calories for a light beer and up to 200 calories for more stout (darker) beers.
- **Wine (4 fluid ounces):** average glass about 100 calories. Remember, some restaurants can be generous with their pouring, so you might be drinking quite a bit more than 100 calories.
- **Mixed and exotic drinks:** A lot of variation here. Your most common drinks range from 150 to 400 calories (per glass), while some of your more exotic drinks can easily have 600-plus calories.

In the back of the book, you will find links to Internet websites that will tell you the approximate number of calories in just about any drink you can think of. I encourage you to explore them and find out how many calories are in your favorite drinks. This way, when you do decide to have a drink or two, you can adjust for it by cutting back on something else in your meal. As the weeks go on and on, your caloric intake charts will get easier and easier to fill out, because as you eat the same things over and over, you will be able to just look at a meal and know how many calories are in it.

Please don't underestimate the importance of counting calories. I know it is tedious. I know it is boring. However, it is crucial that you develop a strong understanding of the caloric content of what you eat. It is the only way to be successful in the long run, unless you plan to stay on the South Beach Diet forever. The good news is that if you think about it, most of us eat the same basic foods day after day, with very little variation. Think about what you have consumed in the last week. If you are eating three meals per day, did you have twenty-one completely, totally different meals last week with no overlap? Probably not.

So ... Get ready ... Get set ... *Start counting!*

Before we move on to the next chapter, let us look at our friend Jane. If you remember, Jane is a forty-year-old woman who is five-foot-five and weighs 170 pounds (BMI = 28).

When we calculated Jane's BMR, we found out that she burns up

1512 calories per day. Realizing this, Jane, trying hard to lose weight, starts a diet that provides her with less than 1500 calories per day. Let's see how she does:

Caloric Intake: Week 1 (Jane)							
Meal	Mon.	Tues.	Wed.	Thurs.	Fri.	Sat.	Sun.
Breakfast	270*	300	400	200	150	500	350
Snack	140	140	220	110	90		120
Lunch	300	409	317	330	310	450	400
Snack		270		140	120		160
Dinner	500	561	400	550	630	670	570
Snack	190		143	90			
Total	1400	1680	1480	1420	1300	1620	1600
				Total Calories for the Week 10,500			

* In order to make this table a little easier to understand, I left out the actual meals and only show the number of calories for each meal.

As you can see, although Jane is eating a reasonably low-calorie diet, it is very hard for her to eat significantly less than her BMR without being hungry all the time. If we just look at how many calories Jane is eating in a week compared to how many calories she is burning up via her BMR:

10,500 Calories IN – 10,584 Calories OUT (BMR, which is 1512 calories / day x 7 days / week) = **–84 calories / week**

So if Jane is negative 84 calories per week, in fifty-two weeks (one year), she will be negative 4368 calories. Remember that one pound of fat is approximately 3500 calories, so she would lose only a little over one pound every year.

$$\frac{-4368 \text{ calories per year}}{3500 \text{ calories per pound of fat}} = \text{weight loss of 1.3 pounds per year.}$$

Luckily for Jane (and the rest of us), our BMR is not the only way we can burn calories. That leads us to the next chapter.

Six

Calculating Your Output

NOW THAT YOU HAVE learned how to calculate your input, you must learn how to calculate your output. The good news is that you have half of this information already. Remember when you calculated your BMR? Add to that your active metabolic rate (AMR), which you will learn about below, and that will give you a good idea of just how many calories you burn up in a day.

Active Metabolic Rate (AMR)

Your active metabolic rate, simply put, is anything that burns calories above and beyond maintaining normal bodily functions.

So, what are some examples of this? Reading, concentrating, walking, running (or any form of exercise) … essentially, anything that is physically or mentally challenging burns extra calories.

Some of these calorie-burning activities are easy to track (such as exercise), and some are not so easy to track (such as studying for a test). For the purposes of weight loss, let us consider your active metabolic rate synonymous with physical activity.

Fat-Burning Foods

There is actually a third component to the output equation, and strangely enough, it is digestion.

I don't think anyone would argue that eating isn't an essential function of life. The number of calories burned during digestion is not considered part of your BMR or your AMR. Nevertheless, it has contributed to another recent and extremely popular (and, unfortunately, totally misunderstood) idea: fat-burning foods.

The term "fat-burning foods" is one that is relatively new to our culture, and one that is starting to appear on more and more food labels.

For example, if you picked up a container of yogurt, it used to say it was the "only yogurt clinically shown to help you burn more fat than cutting calories alone." Reading this statement, one would think that after eating this yogurt, it somehow managed to slip past all the digestive enzymes in your stomach, escape from your intestines, only to travel to your fat cells and start digesting them. That would be some pretty special yogurt!

The only thing that can burn fat is a fire, and let me tell you, if you have ever smelled burning fat, you don't want to go there.

Food manufacturers are not in business to make you healthy, although they would like you to believe that they are. The reason for all of these seemingly helpful manufacturers' labels that tout the merits of their foods with phrases like "low carb," "fat-free," "promotes a healthy heart," "helps burn fat," etc. is that their marketing research has shown them that these labels sell more of their product. Believe me, if their research showed them that putting "smells like crap" on their labels would sell more product, it would be everywhere.

What exactly are these so-called "fat burning" foods then? Taking what goes into your mouth and turning it into something that your body can absorb and then use actually takes some energy (that is, burns calories). And since not all foods are created equal, the amount of energy needed to digest different kinds of foods can vary substantially.

Here's an Example

A small bag of Skittles has about 250 calories. Those 250 calories are derived from 56 grams of carbohydrates (56 grams of carbs x 4 calories / grams = 224 calories) and 2.5 grams of saturated fat (2.5 grams of fat x 9 calories / gram = 24 calories). Of these 56 grams of carbohydrates, 47 grams are just simple sugars. The other 9 grams of carbohydrates are more complex starches, which eventually get broken down into sugars. Now it turns out that your body, from an evolutionary point of view, is pretty well adapted to handle sugar. Since sugar (fructose) is very similar to glucose (a substrate your body can use directly to make energy), very little work needs to be done to get the sugar in Skittles assimilated into your body to be used for energy. It takes your body about 30 calories of work in order to digest and assimilate that 250-calorie bag of Skittles. When all is said and done, you are positive 220 calories.

Now, let's take a quarter-pound of wheat pasta with red sauce. This also has about 250 calories. Again, it is mostly carbohydrates, but this time most of the carbohydrates are complex (not simple sugars). It takes time (and energy) for your body to digest them into the simple sugars it can then absorb. It costs your body about 100 calories to digest and assimilate the pasta. So this time, you are positive only 150 calories for the same 250-calorie meal (for those who consider Skittles a meal).

Meal	1 Bag of Skittles	¼ Cup of Wheat Pasta with Red Sauce
Calories	250 cal	250 cal
Energy Required to Digest and Absorb (in Calories)	30 cal	100 cal
Net Calories	230 cal	150 cal

NOTE: Remember what you've learned. Pasta (when compared to Skittles) takes longer to digest and does not cause a huge insulin spike. Thus, you stay fuller longer and do not get rebound hunger.

Still don't understand why they are called fat-burning foods? Well, to be honest, I don't either. They don't specifically target fat (as explained above). Personally, I think it is just a clever marketing ploy. What it comes down to is that your fat-burning foods are those foods that require more work for your body to digest than others, which burns up calories—and remember, the only thing that will promote weight loss is burning more calories than you are taking in.

For a list of some of the most popular fat-burning foods, please see the back of the book. But remember, just because something is a fat-burning food doesn't mean that you have carte blanche to eat as much as you want. You will still be adding positive calories after eating it, just not as many as if you ate the same number of calories as pure sugar.

Since trying to figure out how many calories you are burning up by eating is be a mind-numbing task (unless you are a biochemist), we are going to assume that the amount of calories you burn up in a day is equal to your BMR plus the number of calories you burn up through exercise, which we will discuss next.

Exercise

In today's society there appears to be a great misconception as to what actually constitutes exercise. Most people seem to think that going for a stroll after breakfast or dinner is exercise. As I say to my patients, that's great, and it is better than sitting at home, but it's not exercise.

Exercise is any type of physical activity that elevates your heart rate over baseline (resting) values. The reason that I specifically say physical activity is because there are many other things that elevate your heart rate, such as mental stress, illness, dehydration, anemia, cocaine, diet pills, and the list goes on and on.

Just as we learned earlier, anything that elevates your heart rate burns more calories, but not to the same degree exercise burn calories. I think just about anyone will agree that trying to lose weight using illness, stress, or one of the other methods mentioned above to increase your heart rate is not a great idea. This is because it is not the increased heart rate that is burning all the calories. Your increased heart rate is just an indicator that your body has an increased metabolic demand. It is this increased metabolic demand—which is due to the repeated contraction and relaxation of thousands of muscle fibers, dilatation and contraction of blood vessels, and hundreds of other bodily processes—that is burning calories.

ATP and ADP, Aerobic and Anaerobic Activity

Adenosine triphosphate, or ATP, is a high-energy chemical compound found in the body that provides the energy that powers virtually every activity of your body—thinking, flexing muscles, talking, etc. ATP works like a rechargeable battery. When ATP is turned into ADP (adenosine diphosphate, or the de-energized form of ATP), energy is released and used to power some cellular process, like causing a muscle fiber to contract. When you eat, many complex chemical reactions occur, but the end result is that you use the energy in food to help your body turn ADP back to ATP to drive more cellular processes.

"Aerobic," a term that most people are familiar with today, and its lesser-known nemesis, "anaerobic," were originally terms used by scientists to describe bacteria. The term "aerobic" was described bacteria that required oxygen to live, while "anaerobic" described bacteria that did not require oxygen to live.

We now use these terms to designate certain types of exercise. Simply stated, aerobic exercise is exercise in which your body primarily relies on oxygen to make ATP, and anaerobic exercise is exercise that doesn't rely on oxygen to make ATP.

Why is this important? Well, it turns out that oxygen is a very efficient way to make ATP, and it is available in limitless quantities (we all hope) in the air we breathe. Therefore, as long as you have stored energy from the food you eat, plus oxygen, you can continually make ATP. Oxygen is also a very clean source of energy, the byproduct being H_2O, or water.

However, if not enough oxygen is available, your body can still make ATP using glycogen. Glycogen is a very complex array of glucose molecules that are stored primarily in your liver and muscles. Unfortunately, glycogen is not as efficient as oxygen in making ATP, and since it is only stored in limited quantities by your body, you eventually run out. Glycogen is also not a very clean fuel source and leaves you lactic acid as a byproduct. This we will discuss in more depth on the following pages.

To look at this in another way, aerobic activity uses oxygen to make ATP, and anaerobic activity uses glycogen to make ATP.

As I said earlier, the key to success in losing weight is doing it for the right reasons: To become a healthier, lighter, and happier you.

The key to a successful exercise program—one that lasts a lifetime— is doing it for the right reasons. Unfortunately, most people who regularly exercise (which, remember, is actually a pretty small percentage of the population), and probably just about all of you who are reading this book, exercise for the wrong reason. The purpose of exercise is not to lose weight. The purpose of exercise is to build a stronger, more metabolically efficient human being.

Here's an Example

Lance Armstrong, who pretty much defines fitness, has a resting heart rate of about thirty-two beats per minute, which is well below the average individual, and even well below most athletes. Why? All of us, when at rest, pump about five liters of blood around our bodies each minute. This is known as your cardiac output. There are two components that make up your cardiac output. The first component is your heart rate. The faster your heart beats or contracts, the quicker it pumps blood.

The second component is called your stroke volume. This is the amount of blood your heart can pump out with each beat. An easy way to think about it is that your heart rate determines the rate at which you pump blood, and your stroke volume determines how much blood you pump with each beat.

$$\text{Cardiac output} = \text{stroke volume} \times \text{heart rate}$$

Remember, your heart is a muscle and, just like any other muscle, it responds to physical stress. Just as when you lift weights, your biceps get bigger and stronger, your heart responds to a slightly different type of stress. This stress is aerobic activity. Again, just as lifting weights can make your biceps more efficient at their job (lifting and moving things), aerobic activity makes your heart stronger at its job of pumping blood.

So through countless hours of aerobic activity, Lance Armstrong's heart has become incredibly efficient at pumping blood. In medical terms, he has a very high stroke volume, or in other words, with each beat, he pumps a lot of blood. As I stated above, at rest, everyone pumps the same volume of blood per minute (cardiac output). If your cardiac output stays the same (five liters per minute in the above example), then your heart rate or stroke volume must change in order to match this. Lance's heart, since he has such a high stroke volume, does not need to beat as often in order to maintain his cardiac output.

Now take someone who has a very small stroke volume; their heart must beat more quickly in order to maintain their cardiac output.

This leads us to your first step in starting a successful lifelong exercise program.

Step 1: Calculate Your Resting Heart Rate (RHR)

Calculating your resting heart rate is easy. Before you go to sleep, put a watch with a second hand, a pad of paper, and a pen or pencil by your bedside table. Now try to locate your pulse—use your wrist and lightly press using your pointer and middle fingers on the thumb side of your wrist. If you do not feel it, move your two fingers slightly up and down or left and right until you find it. You might feel it in more than one place, but what you are looking for is the area with the strongest pulsation. Keep moving your fingers until you are sure you have identified the point of maximum intensity, which will be directly over your artery. Remember to press lightly; otherwise you will temporarily occlude your artery (cut off the flow) and feel no pulse at all.

Once you are confident that you have found your pulse and you can feel it consistently, begin counting the pulsations. When you are comfortable with feeling the pulsations and counting them, try the whole thing over again.

The point here is to be able to quickly find your pulse and accurately count the pulsations. Now try to get a good night's sleep. When you first wake up, before you do or think about anything else, find your pulse and, looking at the second hand on your watch, count how many pulsations you feel for thirty seconds. Multiply that number by two and write it down.

RHR (in beats per minute units) = morning pulse for 30 seconds x 2

Do this again for the next two mornings. You should find that the numbers for all three are pretty similar. If one or two numbers are much different, and you had an unusual morning (for example, if you had a really bad dream right before you awakened, or you woke up because your dog or cat jumped on your stomach), throw these numbers out and take your pulse the following morning. Keep taking your pulse until you have three numbers that are within a few beats of each other. Then add up the numbers and divide the total of the three mornings by three. This is your average resting heart rate.

Average resting heart rate (ARHR) = $\underline{RHR(1) + RHR(2) + RHR(3)}$

Your average resting heart rate will most likely fall somewhere between 45 and 85 beats per minute (bpm). It is very person-dependent and has a lot to do with the effects of the parasympathetic nervous system (which slows down your heart) and the sympathetic nervous system (which speeds up your heart). Some people have a strong parasympathetic system and lower resting heart rates, and others have a stronger sympathetic system and higher resting heart rates.

Also, women tend to have higher resting heart rates than men because they have smaller hearts and smaller stroke volumes. To maintain their cardiac output, their heart rates are slightly faster (remember the Lance Armstrong example).

Your resting heart rate will become a very important number to you, because we will use it to track your fitness progress. We will talk more about this later.

Step 2: Calculate Your Maximum Heart Rate (MHR)

The next thing we need to do is to determine your maximum heart rate. There are two ways to do this. The first way is to *calculate* your maximum heart rate. The second way is to *estimate* your maximum heart rate.

Basically, the way to calculate your maximum heart rate is—after you do your warm-up (on a treadmill or bike)—slowly keep increasing the speed, incline, or resistance on the machine until you are truly at the point of exhaustion. Your heart rate at this point will be your maximum heart rate.

You can try doing this yourself, but it can be very difficult without someone there, like a personal trainer or friend, to motivate you and push you to the point of exhaustion. Also, since your heart will be beating very fast, it will be virtually impossible for you to accurately count your own pulse.

If you do choose to perform a maximum heart rate test by yourself, get a heart rate monitor (HRM) to get an accurate reading. We will talk more about HRMs later.

The way to estimate your maximum heart rate is to use the formula below:

Maximum predicted heart rate (MPHR) = 220 – your age.

Calculate Yours:

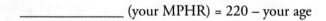 (your MPHR) = 220 – your age

Notice that it is maximum *predicted* heart rate and not maximum heart rate, because it is only an estimate.

Which way is better? The first way, of course, but unless you are a serious athlete, the formula to calculate your MPHR is a good enough place to start. As you become more aerobically fit, you might want to consider professional testing to determine your MHR in order to refine your fitness goals.

Step 3: Calculate Your Target Heart Rate Zones

Using your MHR or MPHR (to simplify things, we will just call it MHR from now on), we are going to calculate your different target heart rate zones. We are going to break your target heart rate into five zones. Please note that all of these numbers are in beats per minute (bpm).

Zone 1 (light activity, like walking.)

Zone 1 is going to be 50 to 60 percent of your MHR. Plug your numbers into the formula below.

____(Your MHR) x 0.5 = ___83_____

____(Your MHR) x 0.6 = ___100_____

Round these values to the nearest whole number. This will give you your heart rate range for zone 1. For example, if your MHR is 183, then your heart rate range for zone 1 will be 92 (0.5 x 183) to 110 (0.6 x 183).

Now fill in the numbers below:

Your zone 1 heart rate range is: ___83___ **to** _100_

Zone 2 (easy activity, like slow jogging.)

Zone 2 is going to be 60 to 70 percent of your MHR. Using the formula below, let's calculate your heart rate range for zone 2.

____(Your MHR) x 0.6 = ___100_____

____(Your MHR) x 0.7 = ___116_____

Your zone 2 heart rate range is: _100_ **to** _116_

As you have probably already noticed, there will be some overlap (i.e. the top number for zone 1 is the same as the bottom number for zone 2. Your heart doesn't understand or care about heart rate zones. They are just artificially derived numbers that we will use to help you understand and obtain your fitness goals.

Zone 3 (aerobic activity. like running.)

Zone 3 is going to be 70 to 80 percent of your MHR. Using the formula below, let's calculate your heart rate range for zone 3.

_____(Your MHR) x 0.7 = ___116___

_____(Your MHR) x 0.8 = ___133___

Your zone 3 heart rate range is: _____ to _____

Zone 4 (anaerobic activity, like running hard)

Zone 4 is going to be 80 to 90 percent of your MHR. Using the formula below, let's calculate your heart rate range for zone 4.

_____(Your MHR) x 0.8 = ___133___

_____(Your MHR) x 0.9 = ___149___

Your zone 4 heart rate range is: _____ to _____

Zone 5 (maximum activity, like running as hard as you can)

Zone 5 is going to be 90 to 100 percent your MHR. Using the formula below, let's calculate your heart rate range for zone 5.

_____(Your MHR) x 0.9 = _____

_____(Your MHR) x 1 = _____
(which is your MHR)

Your zone 5 heart rate range is: _____ to _____

Understanding Your Zones

Now that you have calculated your five zones, let's list them all here for easy reference.

Zone 1: _____ to _____

Zone 2: _____ to _____

Zone 3: _____ to _____

Zone 4: _____ to _____

Zone 5: _____ to _____

Your fitness goals are going to determine which zone you spend most of your time in. Since you are reading this book, I am going to assume that you are trying to lose weight, so we will focus on the zones that maximize weight loss.

Zone 1: This is your "let's go for a walk after dinner" zone, and although this might be a place where many of you have to start (especially if you are really out of shape and haven't exercised for a while), you're not going to burn many more calories than if you stayed at home.

Let's look at an example: a fifty-five-year-old woman with a resting heart rate of 72 bpm. Based on the formula above, her MHR is 165. She will have a heart rate range of 83 to 99 bpm in zone 1. You can see that at the lower end of the zone, she is only 11 beats above her resting heart rate. It is not until she gets to the upper end of zone 1 (closer to zone 2) that you start seeing a more significant increase in her heart rate compared to her resting heart rate.

Remember: the faster your heart pumps, the quicker it can deliver fuel (calories) to your muscles. This fuel is used to make ATP, which drives the contraction and relaxation of your muscles.

Zone 2: In many books and magazines you will see zone 2 nicknamed the fat-burning zone. This is because once you get to above 60 percent of your MHR, your body is very efficiently using energy and oxygen to make ATP to fuel the body.

Zone 3: Also called the "aerobic zone," because it is when your body most efficiently uses oxygen to make ATP to continually contract and relax the muscles. Zone 3 is when your heart learns to become a more efficient pumping mechanism.

Zones 2 and 3 will be your main weight-loss zones. This is because once you get to about 60 to 80 percent of your MHR, your body is very efficiently using energy (burning calories) and oxygen to make ATP as fuel.

Zones 4 and 5: These zones are usually reserved for professional or very serious amateur athletes. Above about 80 percent of your MHR, your heart is pumping so fast that the average person cannot extract enough oxygen from the blood to keep up with the needs of the muscles. When that happens, your muscles turn to glycogen as fuel to make ATP. As we learned above, since glycogen is not as clean as oxygen in making ATP, you get lactate acid as a waste byproduct. Because the lactate acid has nowhere to go, it accumulates in your muscles, causing them to burn.

People work out in these two zones for specific purposes, like trying to push their bodies to make ATP using oxygen rather than glycogen, thus increasing their anaerobic threshold (the maximum heart rate at which you can still efficiently use oxygen as a fuel source). Working out in these zones can also change the types of muscle fibers you utilize—for instance, fast-twitch fibers (which rely on anaerobic metabolism to function) and slow-twitch fibers (which rely on aerobic metabolism to function). For the most part, you will try to stay out of these zones.

Listed in the back of the book are several websites and free programs that will automatically calculate your heart rate zones. Check them out.

Step 4: Exercising with Your New Best Friend

How do you know you which zone you are in? And how do you know that you are staying in your zone?

You can try taking your pulse periodically during exercise by feeling your neck or wrist, but you will soon find that it is very disruptive to your exercise routine, and once you start exercising with some intensity, you will have a hard time finding your pulse and accurately counting it. Most exercise machines today have handles that will display your heart rate anywhere from ten to thirty seconds after you grip them. But again, this tends to be disruptive to your exercise routine, and as your intensity goes up and your heart rate along with it, the grips become less accurate. They tie you to a particular machine (one that has the ability to measure heart rate), limiting the variety you can get in your workouts.

The solution is to buy a heart rate monitor (HRM). This is one of those things that I am going to have to insist on. If you are at all serious about building a stronger, healthier, leaner you, then you need to get an HRM. They have become very popular over the last few years and are the only way to efficiently exercise. They come in many different varieties, so in order to help you make the best decision as to which one is right for you, we will talk about a few.

Probably the gold standard for HRMs are Polar HRMs. A Polar HRM consists of two components: the monitor itself, which essentially is just a watch, and a chest band that senses your heart rate and wirelessly transmits it to the monitor. If it's that simple, then why does Polar have over 20 different HRMs? Like I said, HRMs have become very popular, sellers are trying to cater to individual needs. The reason for the diversity (and difference is price) is all the bells and whistles. On the cheap end (under $50), the Polar FS1 will give you a continuous display of your heart rate while exercising and, after you are done exercising, will show you your total exercise time and average heart rate during that time. It addition to basic watch functions, it will also let you program in your target heart rate zone (i.e., 110 to 123 bpm) and let you know when you are in and out of that zone by beeping.

In the middle-of-the-road range (about $150), is the F11, which, in addition to doing all the above, will also keep track of calories burned, automatically calculate heart rate zones, and keep track of your fitness progress. All of this is downloadable to your computer and can be viewed via Polar's software program, which allows you to display your workouts in graphical format so that you can see what heart rate zone you are spending most of your time in when exercising.

On the high end ($300+), you can get monitors that do a variety of things, such as track the weather, track your speed while running (via satellites), and attach to a bike to give you information such as speed, cadence (revolutions per minute for non-cycling enthusiasts), and altitude.

Which one you choose will depend on the size of your wallet, your ability to learn new gadget skills, and the type of exercise you enjoy the most (if there is one). All of them will get the job done. If I can make a suggestion, try to get one that, in addition to the basic functions, will also tell you the total amount of calories burned during a workout, as this will help you later on.

In the back of the book, I have included website addresses for all the major HRM manufacturers and several online dealers. Shop around and decide which one is best for you.

Step 5: Start Slowly and Aim for the Lower End of Your Zones

When you begin your exercise program, you may notice one of two different bodily responses. If your heart and lungs are in better shape than your muscles, your muscles will give out first, before you can get to your target heart rate. If your muscles are in better shape than your heart and lungs, you will reach your target heart rate very quickly, but won't be able to sustain it for very long. Whichever one of these describes you, just relax and take it slow. Your heart, lungs, and muscles will soon catch up to one another.

When you first start out, aim for the lower part of your target zone. As you get into better shape, slowly build up to the higher part of your target zone. If exercising within your target zone seems too hard, exercise at a pace that is comfortable for you. You will find that with time, you will feel more comfortable exercising and can slowly increase to your target zone.

At first, exercise at a comfortable pace. For example, while jogging or walking briskly, you should be able to hold a conversation. If you do not feel normal again within ten minutes after exercise, you are exercising too hard. As you become more comfortable, you can push your body harder. However, if you ever experience chest pain, feel faint, or have shortness of breath that seems out of proportion for the level of exercise you are doing, go see your doctor.

Step 6: Once You Get Into Your Zone, Do What It Takes To Stay There

Even with all the incredible technology today, man has yet to build a machine as extraordinary as the human body. Its ability to adapt to stress is truly unbelievable. When you lift weights, your muscles get bigger. When you do aerobic exercise, your heart and lungs get stronger, and when you exercise your mind (by learning), your brain forms millions of new neural connections to store this information for a lifetime. I mean, what machine can boast this ability? You may not think so right now, but even your body has this potential. Since your body has this incredible ability to adapt, you must constantly challenge it.

Let us look at an example. Suppose you've decided that you want really big muscles and are going to start a weightlifting program. You are a little short of cash and can only afford to buy a bench and one set of thirty-pound dumbbells. In your exercise routine you do a bench press, shoulder press, bicep curl, and triceps extensions. You do three sets of ten repetitions for each exercise, and that takes you about one hour.

You struggle through the first few workouts, but after a couple of weeks, you can do all three sets of ten repetitions pretty easily. You also notice that your muscles are a little bigger and stronger. You are very happy with your firmer, more toned body and give it another month. However, after the second month, you notice that although your muscles are still firm, they are not getting any bigger. This is because your muscles have adapted. When you first started out, the weight you were lifting was a new stress to your muscles, and this stress caused them to react by getting bigger. But now that they are used to that stress, they don't have as much of a reaction to it.

However, if you then come into a little extra money, buy forty-pound dumbbells, and start using them, your muscles will again react to the new stress (increased weight) by getting bigger.

Well, your heart works in a similar way, except the stress that causes your heart to react is aerobic exercise. Let's say your exercise of choice is the treadmill. When you first start out, you will notice that you will get to your target heart rate zone fairly quickly at a relatively low machine setting. For example, it might take only setting the machine to 2 miles per hour with a 0 percent grade to get you to your target heart rate zone. However, if you do this consistently (at least three to four times per week), you will notice that walking at that same pace (two miles per hour), your heart rate will become lower and lower during the workouts and you may no longer be in your target zone. However, if you change the machine settings (increase the speed or the incline), your heart rate will increase, and then the whole cycle will repeat itself.

This brings up two important points. First, if this is not happening to you, then you are not working out frequently enough or long enough. Your heart needs repetition in order to adapt, just like your brain needs repetition in order to store that information in your long-term memory. Second, once your heart adapts and your heart rate falls out of your zone, it is your signal that you need to push your body harder and get back in your zone.

Step 7: Get Organized

There are many reasons why people fail at achieving their goals, but an important one is lack of organization. Whether it is trying to lose weight, quit smoking, or save money, you need to have a plan to get you there. Starting and sticking to an exercise program is a lot easier if you are organized. First, pick out the times during the week you are going to exercise and put it in your appointment schedule. Think of it just like you would any other appointment. You would not make an appointment to go to the doctor, get a massage, or get a haircut and not go, so why should exercising be any different? Next, make sure you have a specific goal for each workout. For example, "On Wednesday morning at 8 AM, I am going to walk on the treadmill for forty-five minutes, keeping my heart rate between 143 and 152 bpm.

Think about it. If you were a weightlifter, you wouldn't go to the gym, randomly grab different weights, and start doing whatever exercises you thought of first. What if you picked up the first two dumbbells you saw and did biceps curls, then went over to the bench press, put the first two weights you saw on the bar, and started bench-pressing. Imagine how awkward it would feel. It would feel awkward because in order to challenge your muscles to grow, you need to lift weights in an organized and progressive fashion. Remember, your heart is a muscle too, and in order for your heart to grow (and get stronger), it needs to be challenged in an organized and progressive fashion too.

Step 8: Make It Fun

The reason most people don't exercise is because they feel they don't have the time or they don't find exercise enjoyable. When it comes to exercising, you should choose activities that fit your personality and that you enjoy doing. For example, if you like team sports or group activities, then choose things such as basketball, tennis, or aerobics. If you prefer individual activities, choose things such as swimming, jogging, cycling, or walking. Also, plan your activities for a time of day that works best for you. If you are a morning person, exercise before you begin the rest of your day's activities. If you have more energy in the evenings, then plan activities that can be done at the end of the day. You will be more likely to stick to an exercise plan if it is convenient and enjoyable.

Exercising for Maximum Weight Loss

Remember, the primary purpose of exercising is not to lose weight. You should be exercising to help build a stronger, better, healthier person. Having said that, and realizing that being at a healthy body weight does lessen your risk of developing many chronic diseases, we will talk about some ways to exercise for maximum weight loss.

How many calories you burn while exercising is based simply on your weight (it takes energy to move your body around), your heart rate, and time (how long you exercise).

As we discussed earlier regarding your basal metabolic rate, the heavier you are, the more calories you burn. This holds true for exercise too. It takes energy to move the body, and the bigger the body, the more energy it requires. This is another reason why it seems that really fat people can initially lose weight quickly, with even modest exercise. It is because a really fat person has to expend an enormous amount of energy just to move his or her body. Again, the heavier you are, the higher your BMR.

However, as we saw with the BMR, as a heavier person loses weight (and needs to burn fewer calories moving his or her body around), the person's weight-loss plateaus. This phenomenon also holds true with exercising and is a common reason why people who are trying to lose weight stop exercising. They start an exercise program and initially lose weight; that weight loss then slows down or stops, and they get discouraged and quit. However, once again, having read this book and understanding a little bit more about exercise and the human body, you should understand that this is a completely normal phenomenon. Instead of getting discouraged and quitting, you are going to exercise longer and harder and continue to lose weight in order to get that body that you have always wanted.

If you have been really following what I have been saying, you might think, "Why not just get my heart rate as high as possible so I burn off more weight?"

Let's Look at an Example: Lisa and Brenda

Lisa and Brenda are both the same weight. Both want to start an exercise program to become healthier, and secondarily to lose weight. Lisa, who has not read my book, decides to exercise at 90 percent of her maximum heart rate for as long as she can. She initially can go about fifteen minutes before pooping out. Since her workouts are so intense, it takes a while for her muscles to recover. Thus, she can only do them for about three sessions per week. After three weeks, she has increased her exercise time to about twenty minutes per session.

Brenda, who has read my book, decides to put her newfound knowledge to good use. She buys an HRM and decides she is going to exercise at 60 percent of her MHR for as long as she can. Initially, she can go about thirty minutes. When she finishes her workouts, she feels like she has done something, but is not completely drained. This allows her to exercise a little more frequently—five sessions per week. Since Brenda is exercising more frequently and for longer periods, her body is able to adapt more quickly. After three weeks, she has increased her exercise time to 40 minutes per session.

Let's say that Lisa burns 8 calories per minute (cpm) at 90 percent of her MHR.

At week 3, Lisa is burning an additional 480 calories per week (20 minutes x 8 calories per minute x 3 sessions per week).

Brenda burns only half that amount of calories at 70 percent of her MHR (4 cpm).

At week 3, Brenda is burning an additional 800 calories per week (40 minutes x 4 calories per minute x 5 sessions per week).

	Lisa (90% MHR)	Brenda (70% MHR)
Week 1	8 cpm x 15 minutes x 3 sessions/ week = 360 calories/week	4 cpm x 20 minutes x 5 sessions/ week = 400 calories/week
Week 3	8 cpm x 20 minutes x 3 sessions/ week = 480 calories/week	4 cpm x 40 minutes x 5 sessions/ week = 800 calories/week

Who will lose more weight? Brenda will. Although she is exercising at a lower heart rate, she is exercising more frequently and for longer durations. So the key to maximizing weight loss is frequency and duration.

Therefore, what we are going to learn to do is calculate the number of calories burned with aerobic activity. In the back of the book, you will find charts that give the average amount of calories burned for various exercises. These are just estimates and can be used as a rough guide.

For a slightly more accurate way of calculating the number of calories you are burning per exercise, use one of the free energy expenditure formulas available on the Internet (see the back of the book). My advice is to look at a few of them, pick one you like, and stick with it.

However, the best way for you to keep track of the number of calories you burn with exercise is to purchase a heart rate monitor that has that capability—yet another reason to buy an HRM.

Putting All the Exercise Data Together

What we are going to do now is put together an exercise log. This will help you track your progress, show you how much additional energy you are burning, and help you better understand the economics of weight loss.

As an example, let's look at the exercise log for Jane, who we met in Chapter 4.

Exercise Log: Jane, Week 1 (Weight 170 pounds, BMI 28)

Day	RHR	Activity	Total Duration	Average Heart Rate	Calories Burned	Feeling
Mon.	70	Treadmill (3 mph)	35 min.	135 bpm	250	Good
Tues.	71	Nothing				Good
Wed.	76	Treadmill (3 mph)	20 min.	145 bpm	180	Didn't sleep well. Dog barked all night
Thurs.	70	Nothing				Good
Fri.	69	Stationary bike (70 rpm)	45 min.	130 bpm	380	Good
Sat.	72	Nothing				
Sun.	70	Long brisk walk outside (3 mph)	1 hour 30 min.	125 bpm	480	Good

Here is Jane's exercise table after twelve weeks of exercise:

Jane, Week 12 (Weight 160 pounds, BMI 27)

Day	RHR	Activity	Total Duration	Average Heart Rate	Calories Burned	Feeling
Mon.	65	Treadmill (3.0 mph)	45 min.	120 bpm	285	Good
Tues.	66	Nothing				Good
Wed.	64	Elliptical	45 min.	130 bpm	310	Good
Thurs.	65	Nothing				Tired
Fri.	65	Treadmill (3.5 mph)	45 min.	125 bpm	315	Good
Sat.	66	Bicycling (12 mph)	1 hour	130 bpm	410	Good
Sun.	64	Slow run outside (4.5 mph)	30 min.	145 bpm	220	Tired

So, what can we learn from the above tables? The first thing you notice is that Jane's exercise tolerance has gotten better from week 1 to week 12. How do I know that?

Well, first, she is able to exercise longer and more frequently. Second, and most importantly, Jane's average heart rate is lower in week 12 for the same level of exercise.

If you compare both Mondays in which Jane does the same exercise (treadmill at 3 mph), her average heart rate is lower at week 12 than it was in week 1. This is because her heart is adapting to the exercise by becoming a more efficient pump and doesn't need to beat as fast.

You can also tell that her heart is becoming a more efficient pump by comparing her resting heart rates during week 12 to that during week 1. It's about 5 bpm lower. If you remember the Lance Armstrong example, the more efficiently the heart pumps, the less it has to.

A few other things to notice: the longer you work out and the higher your heart rate, the more calories you burn. So make sure you are staying in your heart rate zones, and stay there for as long as you can.

When you are ready to start your own chart, make photocopies of the blank exercise log tables I have provided for you in the back of the book and fill them in.

SEVEN

The Economics of Weight Loss

NOW IT IS TIME to tie it all together. You have been very patient in enduring tedious calculations and formulas, so I will summarize the whole point of this book in one sentence. At the end of the day only one thing matters: that you have burned off more calories than you consumed.

How are you going to know if you are doing that? Yep, you guessed it, another table (This is the last one, I promise.) We are going to title this table "The Bottom Line" and it will look like this:

Week 1: The Bottom Line

Day of the Week	Calories Consumed	Calories Burned (BMR)	Calories Burned (Exercise)	Total Calories Burned	Energy Balance
Mon.					
Tues.					
Weds.					
Thurs.					
Fri.					
Sat.					
Sun.					
Weekly					

NOTE: If you look in the back of the book, you will find that I have provided you with a blank Bottom Line chart. You can make some photocopies of this to help you track your success. The good news is that we already have all the information we need to fill in this table. We just need to find it.

To help you understand how to fill in this last and most important table, we are going to use Jane again as an example. Remember how we had Jane write down everything she ate each day, so that we could see how many calories she was eating with each meal? Go back and look at the caloric intake table we constructed on page 41. We are interested in the last row in that table, which gives us Jane's daily and weekly calorie intake totals. Let's put that information into the first column in the above chart.

Week 1: The Bottom Line

Day of the Week	Calories Consumed	Calories Burned (BMR)	Calories Burned (Exercise)	Total Calories Burned	Energy Balance
Mon.	1400				
Tues.	1680				
Weds.	1580				
Thurs.	1420				
Fri.	1300				
Sat.	1620				
Sun.	1600				
Weekly	10600				

Next, we add in our BMR (calculated in Chapter 4). Remember, the formula we used to calculate your BMR depended on your weight, height and age. You will need to recalculate it as your weight and age change, assuming you are done growing. Small changes in your weight will not have a very dramatic effect on your BMR, so don't drive yourself crazy by continuously recalculating it. I would recommend recalculating every time your weight changes by ten pounds from your baseline.

As we discussed in Chapter 4, Jane is a forty-year-old woman who is five-five and weighs 170 pounds (BMI = 28). Her BMR is 1512 calories per day. Let's say after three months, Jane loses ten pounds and has a birthday. Now she is a forty-one-year-old woman, five-five, weighing 160 (BMI = 26). Her recalculated BMR is about 1460 calories per day. For the purposes of illustration, let's use Jane's original BMR of 1512 calories per day.

Week 1: The Bottom Line

Day of the Week	Calories Consumed	Calories Burned (BMR)	Calories Burned (Exercise)	Total Calories Burned	Energy Balance
Mon.	1400	1512			
Tues.	1680	1512			
Weds.	1580	1512			
Thurs.	1420	1512			
Fri.	1300	1512			
Sat.	1620	1512			
Sun.	1600	1512			
Weekly	10600	10584			

Next, we want to add in the calories Jane burned off with exercise, using from chapter 6 (page 61), Jane's exercise log, week 1, column 6.

Week 1: The Bottom Line

Day of the Week	Calories Consumed	Calories Burned (BMR)	Calories Burned (Exercise)	Total Calories Burned	Energy Balance
Mon.	1400	1512	250		
Tues.	1680	1512			
Weds.	1580	1512	180		
Thurs.	1420	1512			
Fri.	1300	1512	380		
Sat.	1620	1512			
Sun.	1600	1512	480		
Weekly	10600	10584	1290		

Next, add up the calories burned (BMR) and calories burned (exercise), and put that number in the "Total Calories Burned" column. This column will represent your total energy expenditure for each day.

Week 1: The Bottom Line

Day of the Week	Calories Consumed	Calories Burned (BMR)	Calories Burned (Exercise)	Total Calories Burned	Energy Balance
Mon.	1400	1512	250	1762	
Tues.	1680	1512		1512	
Weds.	1580	1512	180	1692	
Thurs.	1420	1512		1512	
Fri.	1300	1512	380	1892	
Sat.	1620	1512		1512	
Sun.	1600	1512	480	1992	
Weekly	10,600	10,584	1290	11,874	

And finally, take the difference between the "Calories Consumed" column and the "Total Calories Burned" column and put this number in the last column called "Energy Balance." As you will see shortly, it is the numbers in this column that will ultimately determine whether you gain, lose, or stay the same weight.

Week 1: The Bottom Line

Day of the Week	Calories Consumed	Calories Burned (BMR)	Calories Burned (Exercise)	Total Calories Burned	Energy Balance
Mon.	1400	1512	250	1762	-362
Tues.	1680	1512		1512	168
Weds.	1580	1512	180	1692	-112
Thurs.	1420	1512		1512	-92
Fri.	1300	1512	380	1892	-592
Sat.	1620	1512		1512	108
Sun.	1600	1512	480	1992	-392
Weekly	10,600	10,584	1290	11,874	-1274

Your energy balance in this last column will be either positive or negative, depending on whether you took in more calories than you burned up, or burned up more calories than you took in. If you burn up (through your BMR and exercise) more than you take in, your energy balance in the last column will be negative. However, if you take in more than you burn up, your energy balance will be positive.

So, what is the point of all this? The point is that at the end of the week, when you add up all the days, you want the number in the lower right-hand corner (weekly energy balance) to be negative; the larger the negative number, the more weight you lose.

The −1274 calories is Jane's energy balance. It is this number that determines whether Jane gains, loses, or stays the same weight.

Again, one pound of fat is about 3500 calories. So if we assume that Jane remains at a −1274 calorie energy balance each week, she should lose about 1.5 pounds per month.

−5096 calorie energy balance each month (-1274 calories / week x 4 weeks / month) ÷ 3500 calories per pound of fat = 1.5 pounds of fat lost each month

I know you're thinking that doesn't seem like a lot, but it is. Losing 1.5 pounds a month is eighteen pounds a year, which is a lot of weight to lose.

But you say, "I don't want to wait a year. What can I do to speed up the process?" That's easy—just look at the table. Your BMR will only get lower as you lose weight and get older, so the only two ways to make your energy balance larger (more negative) is to eat less or exercise more. Let's look at Jane's table from week 12 to illustrate this point.

Bottom Line: Week 12 (Jane)

Day of the Week	Calories Consumed	Calories Burned (BMR)	Calories Burned (Exercise)	Total Calories Burned	Energy Balance
Mon.	1320	1460	285	1745	-425
Tues.	1420	1460		1460	-40
Weds.	1330	1460	310	1770	-440
Thurs.	1430	1460		1460	-30
Fri.	1510	1460	315	1775	-265
Sat.	1450	1460	410	1870	-420
Sun.	1550	1460	220	1680	-130
Weekly	10,010 (wk 1 10,600)	10,220	1540 (wk 1 1290)	11,760	-1750 (wk 1 -1274)

By week 12, Jane has gotten her diet a little more under control and consumes a consistent amount of calories each day. She is eating 590 fewer calories than she did in week 1. She is also exercising longer and more often, burning off an extra 250 calories for the week. However, if you compare her energy balance, she is only negative an extra 476 calories per week. This is because her BMR has changed (gotten lower). I know it seems a little disappointing, but it illustrates two important points. *Weight loss is hard work!* And *it takes time!*

The best thing Jane can do is not to eat less, but to exercise more. She is already consuming a healthy number of calories each day, and by restricting her caloric intake any further (let's say to 900 calories per day), she is going to risk malnutrition and this will cause her BMR to drop, making it even more difficult to lose weight (as in the starvation diet example). She also will likely lose the energy to exercise, which will work against her weight-loss plans.

Let's say Jane really gets into jogging and jogs at a pretty good pace (about 5 mph) for an hour each day, five days per week. An hour of jogging will burn off about 740 calories. So for the week, she is burning up an extra 3700 calories.

If we leave everything else the same from the table for week 12 and just change the amount of calories burned by exercise, something impressive happens.

Week 12: The Bottom Line (with increased exercise)

Day of the Week	Calories Consumed	Calories Burned (BMR)	Calories Burned (Exercise)	Total Calories Burned	Energy Balance
Mon.	1320	1460	740	2200	-880
Tues.	1420	1460	740	2200	-780
Weds.	1330	1460	740	2200	-870
Thurs.	1430	1460		1460	-30
Fri.	1510	1460	740	2200	-690
Sat.	1450	1460	740	2200	-750
Sun.	1550	1460		1460	+90
Weekly	10,010	10220	3700	13,920	-3910

Jane's energy balance is now −3910 calories per week, so she will lose over one pound per week or about five pounds per month. That is about as good as the human body can do. Again, we are talking about *real weight loss.* Not losing water weight or cleaning out your colon, but losing actual fat and keeping it off.

Just remember: nobody is perfect. Everybody splurges, and there is nothing wrong with that. There will be days where you eat more than other days, and there will be days when you don't feel like exercising.

Don't get discouraged; always remember the big picture. At the end of the week, are you negative (in energy balance) or are you positive (in energy balance)?

I promise you this: *If you are eating more calories than you burn off, no matter what diet you are following or what foods you are eating, you will never, ever, ever lose weight.*

So, keep your caloric energy balance negative and eventually you will have the body you have always dreamed of having.

EIGHT

Why Do We Overeat?

IN THE BEGINNING OF the book I touched upon the importance on maintaining a healthy body weight, and in the last few chapters I gave you the tools to do it. I make losing weight sound pretty easy, don't I? *It's not.* Losing weight is one of the hardest things to do. Let me say that again. Losing weight is one of the hardest things to do.

If it were easy, I would not be writing this book. If it were easy, you would not be reading this book. Unlike smoking, or drinking, or drugs you can't just swear off eating for good. Eating is part of life. Without it, there would be no life. Since it is impossible to not eat, we need to teach ourselves to eat responsively.

Eat Responsively

Eating responsively essentially means not overeating and, depending on what your goals are (losing weight, maintaining your weight), eating to achieve those goals. Once again, I have given you a plan for success in the last few chapters; you need to turn that plan into action. Doing so, however, requires a lot more than simply following the steps I have outlined for you.

Eating is more than providing nourishment to your body to sustain life. If eating were only a physical process, it would be easy to tell ourselves, "Stop eating, my body does not need those extra calories." There would be very little thinking at all.

Here is an illustration to help you better understand the issue. When you go to the gas station and fill up your car with gas, what do you do when the nozzle clicks to tell you that your tank is full? You take the nozzle, put it back in the pump, pay for your gas, and leave. You don't think to yourself, "Oh, I wish I could put more gas in the tank." When the tank is full, it's full. The problem is that although the human body may be built like a gas tank, human beings are not. Most of us are not very good at listening to our bodies. It is our minds that call the shots. So when we listen to our minds, eating becomes a very complex behavior with a strong psychological component.

To successfully lose weight, we have to understand and correct the processes that make us overeat in the first place.

I have two dogs, a beagle named Bailey and a Yorkie-poo named Tucson Jack. When I watch the two of them eat I am humbly reminded of how hard it can be to overcome your primal instincts. Bailey, for as long as I can remember, has always dived into his food and kept eating until every drop is gone. Left to his own devices, he literally will eat nonstop until his stomach swells and he is physically sick.

Tucson Jack, on the other hand, eats in a completely different manner. I can put out a full bowl of food for him, and he will eat a little, and when he is no longer hungry, he walks away (at which point Bailey usually comes along and finishes whatever was left).

I realize that no manner of training or discipline is going to change who they are and how they eat. People are not that dissimilar. Human beings, like animals, have a primal instinct to eat. However, there also are a multitude of psychological, genetic, and environmental factors that come into play for each of us when it comes to eating or overeating.

Let us examine some of the most common reasons that people overeat.

Emotional overeating

There are a lot of emotions associated with eating. Some of us overeat when we are happy, some of us overeat when we are sad. There is probably not a single emotion experienced by human beings that does not trigger the response to overeat, in at least someone. Regardless of what initial emotion triggers the urge to overeat, the result is the same. Eating comforts us and makes us feel good.

Let's face it, life is emotional. That is something you can't change, so don't try. What you can change, or at least try to change, is the way you respond to those emotions.

Sit down with a pen and paper and take a good look at your life. Look at all the ups and downs you have experienced and try to remember how you dealt with those situations. Figure out what situations and emotions have triggered you to overeat in the past and be prepared for it next time it happens.

Let's say stress at work has always been a trigger to overeat for you. In the past, whenever you have had a deadline to meet at work you would focus so hard on the task at hand you would not eat all day. However, at some point your primal self (the part of you more interested in self-preservation) would take over and remind you in a not-so-subtle way that you needed to eat, and you would gorge yourself. By the time the week was over and your deadline had passed, you were up five pounds from the repeated cycle of being stuffed or starved.

Next time try planning ahead for your hell week. Go grocery shopping and buy some healthy food and snacks. Then make some healthy meals ahead of time and bring them to work. Now when hell week rolls around and you are completely engrossed in your work, set your watch to beep every three or four hours to remind you it is time to eat something. Grab one of your previously prepared meals or snacks; spend ten or twenty minutes (or however long you can spare) enjoying your food, and get back to work. When the workday is over, if you did things right, you should not be famished. Instead of going home and raiding the refrigerator, head straight to the gym and get in a quick but high-intensity aerobic workup.

I think you will be amazed at how much better healthy eating and exercise are than pigging out as a stress reliever.

Eating to Fit In

Most events in our culture (and probably just about every culture) involve eating and drinking. Unless you are willing to live alone on a desert island, you are not going to be able to avoid the ways in which society functions. Instead of trying to change how society operates, try changing the way you function in society. There is a lot of pressure to eat at parties, dinners, and other social events. No one says that you need to be the wet blanket standing in the corner of the room with a stick of celery and a glass of water in your hand when everybody else is having a good time. Eat. Drink. Enjoy. Just realize that at some point you will need to account for those extra calories you ingested. Whether that means eating less at other meals or doing an extra hour (or two) of cardio, you decide.

Tired of going to social events that revolve around eating and drinking? Here is an idea. Organize your own gathering. A group bike ride, walk, or hike. Throw a different type of dinner party—have everybody cook a low-calorie dish and give out prizes for whoever made the best one. Instead of a band, hire a nutritionist or personal trainer to come talk at your next dinner party. These may sound like crazy ideas, but I think you will probably find that they will be pretty well received. I bet you would be surprised at the number of people who enjoy the social aspects of parties but are also tired of the chronic overeating that goes along with them.

Cultural Overeating

Let me tell you a little about myself. I grew up in New York in a big Italian family. Of course, I love to eat. Many of my fondest memories as a child happened around the dinner table. Every Sunday we would eat until it practically hurt. When I think back I can't say that being stuffed was a good feeling; it was just the way I thought you were supposed to feel after a meal. Eventually as I got older, I stopped forcing myself to eat everything on my plate. Eventually, my Dad did too. It is funny, though. If I ask him why he always ate until he was ready to bust, he tells me that growing up in New York, his parents were so poor that he remembers always walking around hungry. When a good meal came along they ate as much as they could because they didn't know when the next meal would be.

But I did not stuff myself because I was hungry. I did it because it was what I thought I was supposed to do. This is a perfect example of learned behavior (overeating) passed on through the generations. Many cultures are like this. So although overeating may have originally developed out of of necessity (the lack of an abundant food supply), today it is mostly done out of a sense of tradition. I still respect and enjoy my Italian heritage. I love to eat pasta. However, I have modified my habits such that I can enjoy my culture, but eat less.

The Finish-Your-Plate Mentality

Very similar to the cultural overeating that many of us grew up with is the finish-your-plate mentality. When I grew up, one of the rules of the dinner table (besides not throwing food at my sister) was that I would not be not excused from the dinner table until I had eaten everything on my plate. All of us have probably been told at some time or another, "It's a sin to waste food," or "There are starving children in Africa" as a rationale to make sure we ate everything on our plate. These types of remarks have stuck with many of us as adults, and some of us are probably guilty of repeating these statements to our own loved ones. Once again, these statements originated in a time when food was not plentiful, and it is very sad that although we are in the middle of an obesity epidemic in America, there are millions (if not billions) of people in the world who do not have nearly enough to eat.

The reason the finish-your-plate mentality is such a dangerous one has to do with the astronomical increase in portion sizes (see the Supersized America section). Next time you are in a mall, go to the food court. Walk around and look at what people are eating, but more specifically, look at the size of the portions. They are huge! If they don't look too big to you then you truly are a product of twenty-first century America and in need of serious help. The portions today are two, three, even four times bigger than they were even ten years ago. Nevertheless, if you watch people eating, you will notice that most people still clean their plates. It is as if somehow our mind convinces our stomach that whatever amount of food they've put on that plate is exactly how much we should eat. However, just as you have habitually taught yourself to overeat day after day, you can once again teach yourself not to overeat. The key is self control and not necessarily eating everything on your plate.

Compulsive Overeating

Compulsive overeating is the most extreme form of overeating. It is usually characterized by the uncontrollable urge to eat followed by feelings of shame after eating.

Compulsive overeating is emotional eating in its worst form. People who compulsively overeat use food to cope with emotional problems. Whether it is stress, anger, anxiety, fear, depression, or some other psychological distress, compulsive overeaters turn to food to solve their problems. Unfortunately, although food may temporarily alleviate the emotional pain, it does not last, and feelings of guilt and shame for overeating quickly replace the relief.

When we are children, our eating patterns are first formed. Compulsive overeating generally begins at this time. It usually starts in a subtle way. When a child is upset, he or she will be often comforted with food. The child then begins to turn to food whenever upset in order to soothe those upset feelings. Once this pattern of behavior becomes ingrained, it becomes very hard to change, and soon the only way the child knows to deal with emotional problems is by eating.

This behavior follows us into adulthood, and by now other emotional issues have arisen as a result of the compulsive overeating. Feelings such as depression, low self-esteem, helplessness, or lack of control may develop, which in turn leads to more compulsive overeating. It becomes a vicious cycle that is difficult to break.

Sometimes compulsive overeaters will try to gain control over their situation by extreme dieting, diet pills, laxative abuse, or bulimia (recurrent binge eating followed by intentional purging). However, although this may help transiently with weight loss, in the long run it doesn't do anything to remedy—and usually worsens—the emotional reasons for the compulsive overeating.

People who compulsively overeat are often labeled as weak or gluttonous or lacking in self-control. However, with compulsive overeaters, the urge to overeat comes less from our primal side and more from our emotional side. Compulsive overeating is a serious disorder and needs to be dealt with by a health care professional.

Now that we have talked about the psychological aspects of eating and overeating, here are some tips to help prevent you from overeating.

Tips to Prevent Overeating

Cook Less
As I talked about above, many of us have a hard time controlling the urge to finish our plates. One solution is to cook less food. If you cook less the will be less food to eat. It's simple.

Drink a sip of water between each bite

Drinking a sip of water between each bite does several things; it forces you to slow down, it aids in digestion, and it makes you feel fuller faster. Part of the sensation that we are full is a primitive one that has to do with how stretched our stomachs get when eating. When you drink water with your meal, you can eat less and feel just as satisfied, thus cutting out a few extra calories.

Eat slowly

View your meal as a fine wine or a cold glass of beer. Something to be savored. In today's fast-paced world, many of us are guilty of eating on the go or eating so fast that we barely have time to taste the food before it hits our stomachs. This leads to chronic overeating because, by the time your stomach tells your brain that you are full, you have already eaten too much. Eating too fast also deprives you (and your taste buds) of truly enjoying your meal. Make every calorie count by enjoying each bite as much as you can.

Eat as a family

Make mealtime a time to bond as a family. Countless studies have shown that families that eat together have lower rates of both obesity and social and marital problems. Talk about your meal; share with your family or friends the benefits of healthy eating.

Measure out your portions

Along the same lines as cooking less is measuring out your portions. Remember, if you want to truly succeed at losing weight, you need to have an intimate knowledge of how many calories go into your mouth. Know how many calories are in what you are eating and make sure you are eating the appropriate portion size.

Don't pick

Everywhere I look, I see uncounted calories. My office is the perfect example. Chips, candy bars, soft drinks, cookies, doughnuts scattered in every nook and cranny. By the end of the day, they are all gone. However, if I ask one of my coworkers how many calories they ate that day, they always seem to forget to count the little treats scattered around.

Picking or snacking while at work, school, or home is one of the largest yet conveniently ignored sources of extra calories in the average American's diet. We live in a country where there are a lot of tasty snacks to help you make it though the day. I do not think there is a country in the world that comes close to the unbelievable variety of snacks that most of us have grown up with and take for granted.

It is these snacks which have in part created and continue to fuel the obesity epidemic in this country. These snacks are often referred to as empty calories (devoid of nutritional valve), but by watching some people eat them you would think empty calories meant calorie free. I am not telling you to never indulge. All I am saying is that if you are going to indulge in a between-meal snack, you have to count those calories too.

When you eat out, order just an appetizer or split an entrée

Restaurants are in business to make money, not to make you healthy. Unfortunately, it seems that most restaurant owners believe that what keeps people coming back isn't good food but larger and larger portion sizes. Once again, it is hard to resist the urge to not clean your plate, especially when you paying for it. But your health is too important. If there is less food on the table, you will eat less. Make a habit of just ordering an appetizer or splitting an entrée. Even better, insist that the chef cooks only half their normal portion size. Maybe if enough people start doing things like this, the restaurant industry will get the message.

Never feel like you are starving

We covered this earlier, but when you feel like you are starving because your blood sugar has dropped, your more primal side tends to take over, and you are more likely to overeat or make bad food choices.

Never get stuffed

By the time you feel stuffed you have already eaten way too much. Plus, as I mentioned earlier, your body is going to respond to that feeling of being stuffed by over-secreting insulin. You know what happens next: hypoglycemia and the uncontrollable (and primal) urge to, once again, stuff your face with anything and everything.

Bring your lunch and healthy snacks to work

By making your lunch and healthy snacks and bringing them to work, you remain in control. It is easy to get engrossed at work, and next thing you know, you are starving. By packing your own lunch and bringing your own snacks, you can avoid making bad food choices.

Purposely don't finish everything on your plate

Try getting in the habit of not finishing everything on your plate. Put down your fork, push your plate away, and say, "I have had enough." It takes willpower but it can be a liberating experience. Show your primal side who is the boss when it comes to mealtime.

Summary

Even with these tips and the steps outlined in this book, you still only have a slim (no pun intended) chance of succeeding. The simple truth is that historically very few people who try to lose weight succeed. Of those who do succeed, most eventually gain the weight back. Discouraging? Yes, it is. But there are success stories. I see them every day in my office and I am sure that you know a success story or two. The point is that people *are* capable of losing weight and keeping it off. It just takes a good plan of action, a lot of hard work, and the resolve to be able to deal with the myriad of other psychological issues that cause us to overeat.

Also, try to remember, although it may feel like it at times, *food is not your enemy*. Chronic overeating is.

NINE

Your Health and You

I PURPOSELY LEFT THIS section for the end because I don't want to scare you, but to encourage you. However, if I wrote a diet book without addressing some basic health issues, I wouldn't be doing my job.

What should the average American do to have a long, healthy life? The answer to this question is what drew me to cardiology as a specialty. Cardiology, as sophisticated and technical as it can be, is also incredibly simplistic. There are three essential facts: Don't smoke, eat a healthy diet, and exercise.

Now let me ask you. If we have unlocked the secret to living a long and healthy life, why is it that 23 percent of U.S. adults still smoke? Why do 85 percent of U.S. adults not engage in the minimum recommended amount of activity? How come 61 percent of U.S. adults are either over-weight or obese?

Well, there are two basic reasons that I have found: either they are just plain lazy or their priorities are messed up. Believe it or not, for most people, health is not a priority. Most people don't think twice about their health until after something happens. Whether it is that first heart attack (or someone they know having a heart attack), or an abnormal chest X-ray suspicious for lung cancer, most of us start thinking about our health after it is too late.

I am hoping that since you are reading this book, you are either a little more motivated or your priorities are different than your neighbors'. I also hope that after reading this book, you have a better understanding of how to lose weight and exercise. However, I realize now that the one question I have left unanswered is, why?

Why should you lose weight? Why should you exercise? As I touched on earlier in the introduction, most people exercise and diet to improve their appearance rather than for health reasons. So let's put our vanity aside and talk about a few of the reasons why diet and exercise are so important.

Hypertension

Hypertension, or high blood pressure, affects approximately fifty million individuals in the United States and approximately one billion worldwide. The higher your BP, the greater your chance of having a heart attack, heart failure, stroke, or kidney disease. The diagnosis and treatment of high blood pressure are beyond the scope of this book, but for your reference, I have included the most recent hypertension guidelines in the back of the book. These are only guidelines and can change. I encourage you to visit your doctor to have your blood pressure checked. Even if it is only slightly over 120/80, consider making some lifestyle changes. Losing weight, reducing your salt intake, and exercise are among the most effective ways to lower your blood pressure and avoid the need for medications.

High Cholesterol

When doctors say "cholesterol," what they really mean is a fasting lipid profile. Let me explain the difference to you. A total cholesterol test is usually a blood lab test, which is part of a panel of blood chemistry tests (sodium, potassium, etc.). It usually is not a fasting blood sample and gives you a single number, for example, "Total cholesterol = 250mg/dl."

A fasting lipid profile is usually run independently from its own tube of blood and, as the name implies, is done after the patient has fasted for at least eight hours. A fasting lipid profile gives not only your total cholesterol, but also your high-density lipoproteins (HDL), aka "good cholesterol," and triglyceride level. The number for low-density lipoprotein (LDL), aka "bad cholesterol," is actually obtained by the formula LDL = Total cholesterol − HDL − (triglycerides ÷ 5).

The reason for the fasting is that after eating, triglyceride levels temporarily rise. This rise in your triglyceride level causes an underestimation of your LDL. To a cardiologist, a total cholesterol level alone provides only part of the story, and basing treatment decisions on this number alone would be poor doctoring. The number you really want to focus on is your LDL cholesterol. LDL is a major cause of coronary artery disease (buildup of plaque in the arteries of the heart) and heart attacks.

Lifestyle changes, such as reducing your intake of saturated fats and cholesterol, increasing physical activity, and practicing weight control, can dramatically lower your LDL and reduce your chances of developing coronary artery disease and having a heart attack. It is never too early to start. We are detecting coronary artery disease, which used to be thought of as a disease of the elderly, at earlier and earlier ages. With some of the new advances in technology, we are starting to recognize the early stages of coronary artery disease in adolescents and children.

The other number you want to focus on is your HDL cholesterol. This is the number that you want as high as possible. Your HDL is kind of like a scavenger and helps to keep plaque from building up in your arteries. What raises your HDL? Exercising, not smoking, and maintaining a healthy body weight. (I hope you are starting to see a pattern here.)

Again, the diagnosis and treatment of high cholesterol are beyond the scope of this book, but I have included the most current guidelines for cholesterol values in the back. See where you fall. If you have never had a fasting lipid profile and you are over the age of twenty, then it is time to get it checked.

Now to answer the question we asked in Chapter 5: can you develop coronary artery disease if you don't eat any fat?

Yes, you most definitely can.

Like I said earlier, your body needs fat and cholesterol to survive. So even if you eat a low-fat diet (eating a no-fat diet is really not possible), you still can have high cholesterol because your liver has the ability to synthesize cholesterol. So don't assume your cholesterol is okay.

Diabetes

Diabetes is a disease in which the body does not produce or properly use insulin. Insulin is a hormone that is needed to convert sugars, starches, and other foods into energy needed for daily life. Diabetes is the single most important risk factor for developing coronary artery disease. In fact, if you are diabetic, your risk of having a heart attack is the same as someone who has already had a heart attack. Why? There are two main reasons.

First, high blood sugars are a lot like cigarette smoking and somewhat analogous to taking a cheese grater to the inside of your arteries. Both destroy the lining of your arteries, which makes it easier for coronary artery disease to develop. In addition, diabetes keeps bad company. Diabetics tend to have other disorders, such as high cholesterol and high blood pressure, which themselves are risk factors for developing coronary artery disease.

Recently, the number of people with diagnosed diabetes has grown dramatically, not just among older people. The number of children and adolescents who have this disease has increased at an alarming rate. Not coincidentally, the United States is smack dab in the middle of an obesity epidemic. It doesn't take a genius to put two and two together. How do you know if you are at increased risk for developing diabetes? Two things: look at your family and look in the mirror. Diabetes has a very strong genetic component. If you have family members with diabetes, you are at increased risk for getting it yourself. However, there is more to the story.

Look in the mirror. If you are fat, you have an increased risk for developing diabetes. Add a family history of diabetes to some abdominal obesity, and you are almost guaranteed to develop diabetes.

The best way to determine if you have diabetes is with a fasting blood glucose test. A person with a fasting blood glucose level of 126 mg/dl or higher has diabetes.

However, before diabetes, there is "prediabetes." Before they develop diabetes, most people almost always have prediabetes. This is when blood glucose levels are higher than normal, but not yet high enough to be diagnosed as diabetes (between 100 and 125 mg/dl).

The long-term damage that occurs to the body, especially the heart and circulatory system, may already be occurring during prediabetes.

The good news is that although prediabetes and diabetes are serious medical conditions, they can be treated and sometimes cured. By making changes in your diet and increasing your level of physical activity, people with diabetes and prediabetes may even be able to return their blood glucose levels to the normal range. Go see your doctor, get your blood sugar checked, and if it is anything but normal, make some serious lifestyle changes.

So now, why should you lose weight and exercise? Repeat after me: *I want to lose weight and exercise not only to look good, but so I can live a long, healthy and happy life.*

Smoking

No discussion on your health is complete without a few words about smoking. Smoking is America's single most preventable cause of disease and death. What is the second most preventable cause of disease and death? I hope you said obesity.

Each year, smoking leads to 430 thousand deaths and $50 billion in direct medical costs. If that is not enough, lifelong smoking takes an average of ten or twelve years off your life.

Currently about one in four adults (23 percent) are smokers, and, even worse, over one in three adolescents (35 percent) smoke.

Quitting smoking (or even better, never starting) will give you the most bang for your buck. Most people associate smoking with lung cancer. But as a cardiologist, smoking means coronary artery disease or heart attacks to me. The incidence of heart disease in people who smoke is alarmingly higher than those who do not. Cigarette smoking is a recipe for disaster and a short life.

However, cigarette smoking does not stop at the heart. I look at it as an equal opportunity destroyer. It affects all organ systems. If a heart attack does not get you, a multitude of cancers line up to do the job, lung cancer being the most popular one. If you are one of the lucky ones who somehow manages to avoid coronary artery disease and cancer, you have emphysema, stroke, and an increased risk of infection to look forward to. Not to belabor the point any further, but let me emphasize one more time: not smoking is undoubtedly the single most important thing you can do to benefit your health.

How Do I Quit?

There is no one right way, and not every method works for everyone. Get help if you need it. There is a wide array of written materials, programs, and advice to help smokers quit for good. There are many pharmacological and non-pharmacological methods available. Your doctor or dentist is also a good source of help and support. Talk to your doctor. Come up with a plan individualized for you.

Most importantly, *if at first you don't succeed, try, try again.*

CONCLUSION

I NEVER REALLY UNDERSTOOD the point of a conclusion. I mean, what am I concluding, anyway? You, the reader, are the one who has to come to a conclusion. You have read my book. You have understood the information I have presented to you. It is now up to you to make a decision. Ask yourself:

Am I going to be fat for the rest of my life? Or am I going to do what it takes, for however long it takes, to become a healthier, stronger, and happier person?

Don't be mistaken. As a country, America is in the midst of an epidemic—an obesity epidemic. If we don't do something to halt this growing epidemic (no pun intended), we face the very real possibility that for the first time in history, the average American's lifespan may actually start declining. This is how serious the problem of obesity presently is.

As a country, we can change this, but you need to do your part. You may not realize it, but you are a role model for everyone around you. People learn by observing the traits of others. Whether it is your family members, friends, or complete strangers, they are using you as a role model. If you are fat, they think it must be okay for them to be fat.

By following the few simple steps that I have outlined in this book, you have the ability to change and find that skinny person that has been hiding inside you all these years.

You will lose weight and become healthier, not by following ridiculous "dieting secrets" like not eating fruit for two weeks or only eating brown rice instead of white rice. You will lose weight because you are now educated about your body.

You will lose weight because you understand how to make appropriate food choices.

You will lose weight because you understand the importance of aerobic exercise.

And most importantly, you will lose weight because you understand how important it is for your health.

And believe me when I tell you that maintaining a healthy body weight will improve your health and reduce your risks for developing serious illnesses. I'm speaking to you as a cardiologist who sees the sad results of the American obesity epidemic every day. I wrote this book because I want you to understand how critically important it is to keep your weight under control. *You can do it!*

Here's wishing you a happy, healthy, long life.

Salvatore J. Tirrito, MD, FACC

Back of the Book Stuff

Body Mass Index Formula

$$BMI = \frac{Weight\ in\ pounds\ x\ .703}{(height\ in\ inches\ x\ height\ in\ inches)}$$

Calculate Your BMI Online

http://www.nhlbisupport.com/bmi/

BMR Formula

Women

BMR = 655 + (4.35 x weight in pounds) + (4.7 x height in inches) – (4.7 x age in years)

Men

BMR = 66 + (6.23 x weight in pounds) + (12.7 x height in inches) – (6.8 x age in years)

Calculate Your BMR online

http://preventdisease.com/healthtools/articles/bmr.html
http://www.bmi-calculator.net/bmr-calculator

Maximum Predicted Heart Rate Formula

MPHR (or MHR) =220 – your age

Heart Rate Zones

Zone 1: (MHR x 0.5) to (MHR x 0.6) = _____ to _____
Zone 2: (MHR x 0.6) to (MHR x 0.7) = _____ to _____
Zone 3: (MHR x 0.7) to (MHR to 0.8) = _____ to _____
Zone 4: (MHR x .08) to (MHR to 0.9) = _____ to _____
Zone 5: (MHR x .09) to (MHR) = _____ to _____

Calculate Your Heart Rate Zones Online

http://www.heartmonitors.com/zone_calc.htm
http://www.sarkproducts.com/targetzonecalculator.htm
http://www.freedieting.com/tools/target_heart_rate.htm
http://www.machinehead-software.co.uk/bike/heart_rate/heart_
rate_calculator.html (free downloadable program that will calculate your MPHR and zones by several different (and well-validated)
methods

Buying a Heart Rate Monitor

Here are some great sites to buy an HRM online. They carry all the major brands:

- http://www.heartratemonitorsusa.com/index.html
- http://www.everythingfitness.com/heart-rate-monitors.html
- http://www.heartmonitors.com

Individual HRM Company Websites

Polar: http://www.polarusa.com

Cardiosport: http://www.cardiosport.com

Reebok: http://store.reebok.com/home/index.jsp

Timex: http://www.timex.com

Garmin: http://www.garmin.com

Sports Instruments: http://www.sportsinstruments.com

Sportline: http://www.walkingadvantage.com

Impact Sports: http://www.impactsports.com (really neat alterna-
tive for those people who won't wear a strap)

Mio: http://www.miowatch.com

Calculating Calories Burned with Various Exercises

Websites

http://www.coolnurse.com/calories.htm

http://preventdisease.com/healthtools/articles/various_sports.html

http://www.annecollins.com/weight_loss_tips/calories.htm

Tables

This table lists a wide variety of exercises and the average caloric expenditures for a 125-pound woman and a 170-pound man for ten minutes of exercise.

Activity and Calories/10 minute	125-lb Woman	170-lb Man
Basketball	77	106
Cycling (5.5 mph)	36	49
Cycling (9.4 mph)	56	74
Cycling (racing)	95	130
Dance exercise (high-impact aerobics)	94	124
Dance exercise (low-impact aerobics)	80	105
Football	74	102
Racquetball	76	107
Rope skipping (slow)	82	116
Rope skipping (fast)	100	142
Running (8 minutes/mile)	113	150
Running (11½ min/mile)	76	100
Skiing (cross-country)	80	106
Stairmaster	88	122
Step aerobics (4-inch bench)	48	66
Step aerobics (6-inch bench)	58	80
Step aerobics (8-inch bench)	67	92
Step aerobics (10-inch bench)	75	104
Soccer	78	107
Swimming (backstroke)	95	130
Swimming (breaststroke)	91	125
Swimming (fast crawl)	87	120
Swimming (slow crawl)	95	130
Swimming (sidestroke)	68	90
Swimming (treading water)	35	48
Tennis (singles)	61	81
Volleyball	28	39
Weight training (super circuit)	104	137
Weight training (muscular strength)	44	60
Weight training (muscular endurance)	58	80
Walking (3.5 mph)	45	59

In the following table, Calories are given for one minute of activity. To determine approximately how many calories you burn in half an hour, find the number for your activity and weight, then multiply that number by 30.

Activity and Calories/minute	120 lb	140 lb	160 lb	180 lb
Aerobics (traditional)	7.4	8.6	9.8	11.1
Basketball	7.5	8.8	10.0	11.3
Bowling	1.2	1.4	1.6	1.9
Cycling (10 mph)	5.5	6.4	7.3	8.2
Golf (pull/carry clubs)	4.6	5.4	6.2	7.0
Golf (power cart)	2.1	2.5	2.8	3.2
Hiking	4.5	5.2	6.0	6.7
Jogging	9.3	10.8	12.4	13.9
Running	11.4	13.2	15.1	17.0
Sitting quietly	1.2	1.3	1.5	1.7
Skating (ice and roller)	5.9	6.9	7.9	8.8
Skiing (cross-country)	7.5	8.8	10.0	11.3
Skiing (downhill and water)	5.7	6.6	7.6	8.5
Swimming (crawl and moderate pace)	7.8	9.0	10.3	11.6
Tennis	6.0	6.9	7.9	8.9
Walking	6.5	7.6	8.7	9.7

Calorie Requirement in Kilocalories by Gender and Age

Activity Level (a, b, c)				
Gender	Age (Years)	Sentary[a]	Moderately Active[b]	Active[c]
Child	2–3	1,000	1,000–1,400	1,000–1,400
Female	4–8	1,200	1,400–1,600	1,400–1,800
	9–13	1,600	1,600–2,000	1,800–2,200
	14–18	1,800	2,000	2,400
	19–30	2,000	2,000–2,200	2,400
	31–50	1,800	2,000	2,200
	51+	1,600	1,800	2,000–2,200
Male	4–8	1,400	1,400–1,600	1,600–2,000
	9–13	1,800	1,800–2,200	2,000–2,600
	14–18	2,200	2,400–2,800	2,800–3,200
	19–30	2,400	2,600–2,800	3,000
	31–50	2,200	2,400–2,600	2,800–3,000
	51+	2,000	2,200–2,400	2,400–2,800

a. "Sedentary" means a lifestyle that includes only the light physical activity associated with typical day-to-day life.

b. "Moderately active" means a lifestyle that includes physical activity equivalent to walking about 1.5 to three miles per day at 3 to 4 miles per hour, in addition to the light physical activity associated with typical day-to-day life

c. "Active" means a lifestyle that includes physical activity equivalent to walking more than three miles per day at 3 to 4 miles per hour, in addition to the light physical activity associated with typical day-to-day life.

Great Sites that Educate You on General Health and Nutrition

- http://www.drheartwise.com

- http://www.americanheart.org

- http://www.cdc.gov

- http://health.nih.gov

- http://www.abouthypertension.info

- http://www.diabetes.org/home.jsp

- http://www.nutrition.gov

- http://www.nhlbi.nih.gov/guidelines/cholesterol/atp_iii.htm

- http://www.acefitness.org

- http://www.nhlbi.nih.gov/guidelines/hypertension/jncintro.htm

- http://www.caloriesperhour.com/tutorial_ideal.html

- http://www.healthierus.gov/dietaryguidelines

Protein Facts

According to official U.S. guidelines, the recommended daily allowance (RDA) of protein for adults is 0.8 gram per kilogram (2.2 pounds) of ideal body weight. The following tables show the nutritional content of various high protein content foods.

Beef	Quantity	Calories	Fat	Protein
Round, top, lean, raw	1 lb	576	15g	103.5g
Round, bottom, lean, raw	1 lb	653	25.5g	99g
Round, top, raw	1 lb	798.5	42.5g	97.5g
Chuck, arm pot roast, lean, raw	1 lb	589.5	20g	96.5g
Round, tip, lean, raw	1 lb	562.5	17.5g	96.5g
Top sirloin, lean, raw	1 lb	589.5	20g	96.5g
Pork	**Quantity**	**Calories**	**FAT**	**Protein**
Pork loin, whole, lean, raw	1 lb	648.5	25.5g	97g
Pork sirloin (chops/roast), bone-in, lean, raw	1 lb	644	26g	95.5g
Pork tenderloin, lean, raw	1 lb	544.5	15.5g	95g
Ham, whole, lean, raw	1 lb	617	24.5g	93g
Chicken	**Quantity**	**Calories**	**FAT**	**Protein**
Chicken meat and skin , fried batter	1 lb chicken	809	48.5g	63g
Chicken meat and skin , roasted	1 lb chicken	425.5	24g	48.5g
Turkey meat and skin, roasted	1 lb turkey	499	23.5g	67.5g
Turkey meat only, roasted	1 lb turkey	353.5	10.5g	61g
Fish	**Quantity**	**Calories**	**FAT**	**Protein**
Grouper fish, mixed species	1 fillet (259g)	238.5	2.5g	50g
Mackerel fish, Pacific and Jack	1 fillet (225g)	355.5	18g	45g
Red snapper fish, mixed species	1 fillet (218g)	218	3g	44.5g
Salmon fish , coho, wild	½ fillet (198g)	289	11.5g	43g
Halibut fish , Atlantic and Pacific	½ fillet (204g)	224.5	4.5g	42.5g
Vegetables	**Quantity**	**Calories**	**FAT**	**Protein**
Kidney beans	1 cup	612	1.5	43g
Chickpeas	1 cup	728	12g	38.5g
Lima beans	1 cup	601	1g	38g
Soy beans	1 cup	376	17g	33g
Nuts	**Quantity**	**Calories**	**FAT**	**Protein**
Butternuts, dried nuts	1 oz	173.5	16g	17g
Peanut butter with salt	2 Tbsp	190	16.5g	8g
Pine nuts, pignolia, dried nuts	1 oz	160.5	14.5g	7g
Walnuts, black, dried nuts	1 oz	172	16g	7g

Nutrient Content of Selected Dairy Foods

Product	Serving Size	Calories	Protein (g)	Carbs (g)	Fat (g)	Calcium (mg)
Milk						
Whole	1 cup	150	8	11.4	8.2	291
Reduced fat	1 cup	121	8.1	11.7	4.7	297
Low fat	1 cup	104	8.5	12.2	2.4	313
Nonfat	1 cup	90	8.8	12.3	0.6	316
Chocolate, Whole	1 cup	208	7.9	25.9	8.5	280
Chocolate, reduced fat	1 cup	179	8	26	5	284
Chocolate, low fat	1 cup	158	8.1	26.1	2.5	287
Cheese						
Cheddar	1 oz	114	7	0.4	9.4	204
Cream	1 oz	99	2.1	0.8	9.9	23
Mozzarella, Part Skim	1 oz	79	7.8	0.9	4.9	207
American/ Pasteurized Processed	1 oz	106	6.3	0.5	8.9	174
Cottage	1 cup	82<	14	3.1	1.1	69
Yogurt						
Whole Milk	1 cup	150	8.5	11.4	8	296
Nonfat	1 cup	137	14	18.8	0.4	488

Carbohydrate Facts

Unfortunately, in today's society carbohydrates have gotten a bad rap. In actuality, the bulk of your daily calories should come from carbohydrates (45 to 65 percent). It is also recommended that you have 14 grams of fiber for every 1000 calories consumed

Complex Carbs

- Legumes, such as lentils, peas, and beans
- Vegetables, such as beets, broccoli, cabbage, carrots, cauliflower, corn, lettuce, peppers, potatoes
- Grains, nuts, and seeds, including whole-grain bread, pasta, cereal, and flour

Refined Carbs

- Most unsweetened, but refined (non-whole-grain)
- Cereal
- Bread
- Granola
- Pasta
- Baked goods

Simple Carbs

- Candy
- Honey
- Pop
- Donuts
- Sweetened cereal
- Cakes
- Sweet fruits, fruit juice
- White sugar, brown sugar, corn syrup, maple syrup, molasses, sucrose, glucose, fructose, dextrose, and other variationsGlycemic Index of Various Foods

Low-GI Foods

All-Bran

Apples

Apple juice

Apricots, dried

Artichoke

Asparagus

Baked beans, canned

Banana

Banana bread

Broccoli

Bulgur

Carrots, cooked

Cauliflower

Celery

Cherries

Chickpeas, canned

Chocolate bar, 1.5 oz

Cucumber

Custard

Eggplant

Fettuccine

Grapefruit

Grapefruit juice

Grapes

Green beans

Green peas

Ice cream, low-fat

Kidney beans, canned

Kiwifruit

Lentil soup, canned

Lettuce, all varieties

Lima beans, baby frozen

Macaroni

Mars, Snickers Bar

Milk, fat-free

Oat bran bread

Oatmeal, old-fashioned

Orange juice, not from concentrate

Oranges

Peaches

Peaches, canned natural juice

Peanuts

Peanut M&Ms

Pearled barley

Pears

Peas, dried

Peppers, all varieties

Pineapple juice

Pinto beans, canned

Plum

Potato chips

Pound cake

Rice, parboiled

Rice, long-grain

Snow peas

Spaghetti

Spaghetti, whole wheat

Special K

Spinach

Soy milk

Sweet potato

Tomatoes

Tomato soup

Tortellini, cheese

Yogurt, low-fat, artificially sweetened

Yogurt, low-fat, sweetened with sugar

Zucchini

Intermediate-GI Foods

Angel food cake
Apricots, canned light syrup
Beets
Black bean soup, canned
Blueberry muffin
Bran Chex
Bran muffin
Bread, rye American
Bread, rye crisp
Bread, white
Bread, whole wheat
Corn, sweet
Couscous
Fruit cocktail, canned
Grape-Nuts
Green pea soup, canned
Hamburger bun
Ice cream
Kudos
Life Savers
Linguine

Macaroni and cheese
Melba toast
Mini shredded wheat
Muesli
Oatmeal cookies
Oatmeal, instant
Oatmeal, quick-cooking
Orange juice, frozen concentrate
Peaches, canned, heavy syrup
Pineapple
Pita bread
Pizza, cheese
Popcorn
Raisins
Rice, brown
Rice, white
Stoned Wheat Thins
Sugar (sucrose), table
Taco shells
Whole grain bars (chocolate chip)

High-GI Foods

Bagel

Bread, french

Bread stuffing mix

Cheerios

Corn Chex

Corn chips

Cornflakes

Cream of Wheat instant

Dates

Doughnuts

French fries

Frozen waffles

Golden Grahams

Graham crackers

Grape-Nuts Flakes

Jelly beans

Parsnips

Potatoes, baked

Potatoes, mashed

Potatoes, mashed, instant

Pretzels

Puffed wheat

Rice cakes

Rice Chex

Rice, instant

Rice Krispies

Roll, honey, Kaiser

Total cereal

Vanilla wafers

Watermelon

Fat Facts

Consume less than 10 percent of calories from saturated fatty acids and less than 300 mg per day of cholesterol, keeping trans fatty acid consumption as low as possible. Keep total fat intake between 20 to 35 percent of calories, with most fats coming from sources of polyunsaturated and monounsaturated fatty acids, such as fish, nuts, and vegetable oils.

You can make lower-fat, healthier food choices and still enjoy your meals. The key is moderation. Also, try to choose the lower-fat versions of everyday foods. Instead of eating fatty flank steak, try leaner rib eye. Try drinking low-fat or skim milk rather than whole milk. When cooking chicken, take the skin off. Try baking fish rather than frying it. The chart on the following page will help you learn to make healthier choices. Use it daily and you just might be surprised at the results. You might also be surprised that you don't miss that extra fat (and calories) at all.

	High-Fat Foods		Lower-Fat Alternatives
Beef	Rib roasts Hamburger Rib-eye sirloin and T-bone	→	Extra lean ground beef Flank steak, sirloin tip Round steak.
Pork	Shoulder cuts Sausages Lunch meats	→	Loin chops Fresh/smoked ham Pork tenderloin
Chicken	With skin, fried	→	Without skin. broiled, baked, or grilled
Seafood	Breaded and fried	→	Grilled, broiled, or baked
Cheese	Cheddar American Bleu Swiss	→	Part skim Mozzarella Parmesan
Cereal, Grains	Granola	→	Oatmeal Cornflakes Cheerios Shredded Wheat Puffed rice
Potatoes	French fries Au gratin	→	Oven-fried Baked
Salad Dressing	Regular salad dressings	→	Low-cal salad dressings
Snack Foods	Peanuts Potato chips Cheese Curls Tortilla chips	→	Unbuttered popcorn Pretzels Rice cakes
Cake	Layer or pound	→	Angel food or sponge
Ice Cream	Ice cream	→	Frozen yogurt

"Fat-Burning Foods"

Remember again why they are called fat-burning foods. It is not because they somehow magically dissolve fat; it is because they take more energy to digest (compared to non-fat-burning foods like simple sugars), which means you are burning more calories.

Apples	Eggplant	Peaches
Apricots	Flounder	Pears
Artichokes	Garlic	Peas
Asparagus	Grapefruit	Peppers
Beets	Grapes	Pineapple
Blackberries	Green beans	Prunes
Blueberries	Honeydew	Pumpkin
Broccoli	Kale	Radishes
Brussels sprouts	Leeks	Raspberries
Cabbage	Lemon	Red cabbage
Cantaloupe	Lettuce	Sauerkraut
Carrots	Limes	Scallions
Cauliflower	Lobster	Spinach
Celery	Mangoes	Squash
Cherries	Milk	Strawberries
Cheeses	Mushrooms	String beans
Chives	Nectarines	Tangerines
Cod	Okra	Tomatoes
Corn	Onions	Turnips
Crabs	Oranges	Watermelon
Cranberries	Papaya	Yogurt
Cucumbers	Parsley	

Websites to Help You Succeed

Calories in Alcoholic Mixed Drinks

http://www.dietbites.com/calories/calories-in-alcohol.html

Calories in Beer

http://www.beer100.com/beercalories.htm

Calories in Various Foods and Snacks (General)

http://www.calorie-count.com/calories

Calories in Wine

http://www.annecollins.com/calories/calories-wine.htm

Frito-Lay Snack Products Nutritional Info

http://www.fritolay.com/fl/flstore/cgi-bin/products.htm

Fast-Food Chain Stores Nutritional Info

(Please note some of these link to Adobe PDF files. In order to view them, you will need to have Adobe Acrobat Reader installed on your computer. You can get it free at http://www.adobe.com).

Arby's: http://www.arbys.com/nutrition/printable. php?type=nutrition

Baja Fresh: http://www.bajafresh.com/nutritional.php

Baskin-Robbins: http://www.baskinrobbins.com/Nutrition

Ben & Jerry's: http://www.benjerry.com/our_products/nutritional_ info_all.cfm

Blimpie: http:// http://blimpiebirthday.kahalacorp.com/na/index. php

Burger King: http://www.bk.com/Nutrition/PDFs/brochure.pdf

Caribou Coffee: http://www.cariboucoffee.com/menu/ nutritioninfo.asp

Carl's Junior: http://www.carlsjr.com/content/downloads/nutrition.pdf

Chick fil-A: http://www.chickfila.com/documents/NutritionalInfo.pdf

Chipotle: http://www.chipotle.com/images/nutrition.pdf

Church's Chicken: http://www.churchs.com

CiCi's Pizza: http://www.cicispizza.com/Menus_Nutrition.asp

Cold Stone Creamery: http://www.coldstonecreamery.com/secondary/news5.asp

Dairy Queen: http://www.dairyqueen.com/us-en/eats-and-treats/nutrition-calculator

Domino'shttp://www.dominos.com/home/menu/nutritional.jsp

Dunkin Donuts: https://www.dunkindonuts.com/aboutus/nutrition

Einstein Bros:http://www.einsteinbros.com/pdf/nutrition_info.pdf

Fazoli's: http://fazolis.com/menu/nutritional_information.aspx

In-N-Out Burger: http://www.in-n-out.com/nutritional_info.asp

Jack in the Box: http://www.jackinthebox.com/ourfood

Jamba Juice: http://www.jambajuice.com/menuguide

Jason's Deli: Email nutrition requests to nutrition@jasonsdeli.com

KFC: http://www.yum.com/nutrition/documents/kfc_nutrition.pdf

Krispy Kreme: http://www.krispykreme.com/nutri2.html

Krystal: http://www.krystal.com/Krystal_Nutrition_Facts.pdf

Little Caesar's: http://www.littlecaesars.com/menu/nutrition.asp

McDonalds: http://www.mcdonalds.com/app_controller.nutrition.index1.html

Noodles and Company: http://www.noodles.com/menu_diet_guide.asp

Papa John's: http://www.papajohns.com/menu/index.htm

Pizza Hut: http://www.pizzahut.com/menu/nutritioninfo.asp

Planet Smoothie: http://planetsmoothie.com/smoothie-nutrition.php

Popeye's: http://www.popeyes.com/nutrition

Quizno's: http://www.quiznos.com/menu/nutrition.asp

Sbarro: http://www.sbarro.com/ourFood/nutrition.php

Schlotzky's: http://www.schlotzskys.com/nutrition.html

Smoothie King: http://www.smoothieking.com

Sonic: http://www.sonicdrivein.com/pdfs/menu/SonicNutritionGuide.pdf

Starbucks: http://www.starbucks.com/retail/nutrition_info.asp

Steak n Shake: http://www.steaknshake.com/nutritional_info/nutricalc/index.asp

Subway: http://www.subway.com/applications/NutritionInfo/index.aspx

Taco Bell: http://www.yum.com/nutrition/documents/tb_nutrition.pdf

Wendy's: http://www.wendys.com/food/pdf/us/nutrition.pdf

White Castle: http://www.whitecastle.com/_pages/nutrition.asp

Wienerschnitzel: http://www.wienerschnitzel.com/wiener/ourfood/nutrition_new.pdf

Whataburger: http://www.whataburger.com/menulist.cfm

Tables and Charts to Help You Succeed

Body Weight in Pounds According to Height and Body Mass Index														
BMI (kg/m2)	19	20	21	22	23	24	25	26	27	28	29	30	35	40
Height (inches)	Weight (lb)													
58	91	96	100	105	110	115	119	124	129	134	138	143	167	191
59	94	99	104	109	114	119	124	128	133	138	143	148	173	198
60	97	102	107	112	118	123	128	133	138	143	148	153	179	204
61	100	106	111	116	122	127	132	137	143	148	153	158	185	211
62	104	109	115	120	126	131	136	142	147	153	158	164	191	218
63	107	113	118	124	130	135	141	146	152	158	163	169	197	225
64	110	116	122	128	134	140	145	151	157	163	169	174	204	232
65	114	120	126	132	138	144	150	156	162	168	174	180	210	240
66	118	124	130	136	142	148	155	161	167	173	179	186	216	247
67	121	127	134	140	146	153	159	166	172	178	185	191	223	255
68	125	131	138	144	151	158	164	171	177	184	190	197	230	262
69	128	135	142	149	155	162	169	176	182	189	196	203	236	270
70	132	139	146	153	160	167	174	181	188	195	202	207	243	278
71	136	143	150	157	165	172	179	186	193	200	208	215	250	286
72	140	147	154	162	169	177	184	191	199	206	213	221	258	294
73	144	151	159	166	174	182	189	197	204	212	219	227	265	302
74	148	155	163	171	179	186	194	202	210	218	225	233	272	311
75	152	160	168	176	184	192	200	208	216	224	232	240	279	319
76	156	164	172	180	189	197	205	213	221	230	238	246	287	328

Risk of Associated Disease According to BMI and Waist Size			
BMI		Waist Less Than or Equal to 40 inches (Men) or 35 inches (Women)	Waist Greater Than 40 inches (Men) or 35 inches (Women)
18.5 or Less	Underweight	—	N/A
18.5–24.9	Normal	—	N/A
25.0–29.9	Overweight	Increased	High
30.0–34.9	Obese	High	Very high
35.0–39.9	Obese	Very high	Very high
40 or Greater	Extremely obese	Extremely high	Extremely high

JNC 7 Classification of Blood Pressure for Adults Over Eighteen Years Old

CATEGORY		Systolic Blood Pressure (mm Hg)		Diastolic Blood Pressure (mm Hg)
Normal		<120	and	<80
Pre-Hypertension		120–139	or	80–89
	Stage I	140–159	or	90–99
	Stage II	>160	or	≥100

The Seventh Report of the Joint National Committee on Prevention, Detection, Evaluation, and Treatment of High Blood Pressure. Bethesda, MD. National Institutes of Health, National Heart, Lung, and Blood Institute. 2003; NIH Publication 03-5231.

The above chart applies to people not taking antihypertensive drugs and who are not acutely ill. When systolic and diastolic pressures fall into different categories, the higher category should be selected to classify the individual's blood pressure status.

ATP III Classification of LDL Cholesterol, Total Cholesterol, HDL Cholesterol, and Triglycerides (mg/dL)

LDL Cholesterol - Primary Target of Therapy

<100	Optimal
100–129	Near/above optimal
130–159	Borderline high
160–189	High
>190	Very high

Total Cholesterol

<200	Desirable
200–239	Borderline high
>240	High

HDL Cholesterol

<40	Low
>60	High

Triglycerides

<150	Normal
150–199	Borderline high
200–499	High
>500	Very high

PDF versions of the following charts can be found and downloaded from www.drheartwise.com.

| Caloric Intake: Week _____ | | | | | |
Meal	Monday	Tuesday	Wednesday	Thursday	Friday
Breakfast					
Snack					
Lunch					
Snack					
Dinner					
Snack					
Total					
			TOTAL CALORIES FOR THE WEEK_____		

Exercise Log: Week _____

Day of the Week	RHR	Activity	Total Duration	Average HR	Total Calories Burned	Feeling
Monday						
Tuesday						
Wednesday						
Thursday						
Friday						
Saturday						
Sunday						
			TOTAL CALORIES BURNED FOR THE WEEK_____			

The Bottom Line: Week _____					
Day of the Week	Calories Consumed	Calories Burned (BMR)	Calories Burned (Exercise)	Total Calories Burned	Energy Balance
Monday					
Tuesday					
Wednesday					
Thursday					
Friday					
Saturday					
Sunday					
Weekly					